CHARCOT-MARIE-TOOTH DISORDERS:

A Handbook for Primary Care Physicians

Editor
Gareth J. Parry, MD, FRACP
Department of Neurology
University of Minnesota
Minneapolis, Minnesota

The publication of this book was supported by a grant from Athena Diagnostics, a division of Athena Neurosciences, Inc.

Charcot-Marie-Tooth Association
Upland, PA

All correspondence and inquiries should be directed to
The Charcot-Marie-Tooth Association,
601 Upland Avenue, Upland, PA 19015

ISBN: 0-7881-1528-6

Printed in the United States of America

To Dr. Robert E. Lovelace

physician, teacher, scientist
without whose inspiration this volume would not have been accomplished.

CHARCOT-MARIE-TOOTH DISORDERS: A Handbook for Primary Care Physicians

Contents

CHARCOT-MARIE-TOOTH DISEASE HISTORICAL PERSPECTIVE AND OVERVIEW

Professor P.K. Thomas, CBE, MD, DSc FRCP

Royal Free Hospital
School of Medicine and Institute of Neurology
London, UK

Key words: *hypertrophic neuropathy, onion bulbs, demyelination, Roussy-Levy syndrome, Fredreich's ataxia, spinal muscular atrophy, prevalence, genetic counseling, foot care, peroneal muscular atrophy*

The peroneal type of muscular atrophy was separated from other forms of progressive neuromuscular disorders in 1886, simultaneously by Charcot and Marie in France and Tooth in the UK. Very shortly afterwards, Dejerine and Sottas, again in France, identified cases of hereditary neuropathy in which the characteristic feature was considered to be the presence of an intriguing type of morphologic change in the peripheral nerves referred to as an interstitial hypertrophic neuropathy of "onion bulb" type. The nerve fibers were surrounded by concentrically proliferated cells resembling a cross-section of an onion. This was initially believed to represent a specific entity, Dejerine-Sottas disease or hereditary hypertrophic neuropathy, in which the peripheral nerves were markedly thickened.

The salient clinical feature of the patients described by Charcot, Marie, and Tooth was an hereditary disorder giving rise to distal limb weakness, maximal in the lower extremities (peroneal muscular atrophy), commonly with an onset in childhood and adolescence and frequently associated with foot deformity. Tendon areflexia was frequent and there was variable distal sensory loss. The disorder was only slowly progressive.

The situation became increasingly confused when variants of this pattern were described, such as the Roussy-Lévy syndrome that combined familial claw foot, ataxia, and tendon areflexia. It was often considered to represent an intermediate condition in a spectrum between peroneal muscular atrophy and Friedreich's ataxia. Hypertrophic changes in peripheral nerves were found in patients with typical peroneal muscular atrophy (Hoffmann's syndrome). They were also found in Refsum's syndrome, an inherited neuropathy resulting from low phytanic acid, once this was identified as a separate entity. Identification of hypertrophic changes in many different inherited neuropathies called into question the status of Dejerine-Sottas disease as a discrete condition.

The first semblance of order emerged in 1968, in a study by P.J. Dyck and E.H. Lambert made possible by the introduction of nerve conduction studies into the clinical realm and advances in the understanding of peripheral nerve pathology. Shortly before this, it had been established that hypertrophic neuropathy was not a specific process but the nonspecific consequence of repeated episodes of demyelination and remyelination.

Dyck and Lambert showed that some patients with a clinical diagnosis of peroneal muscular atrophy or Charcot-Marie-Tooth disease had a purely motor syndrome. These are now generally designated as distal spinal muscular atrophy. The remainder had additional involvement of the primary sensory neurons, hence the fact that these examples of Charcot-Marie-Tooth (CMT) disease are often referred to by neurologists as hereditary motor and sensory neuropathy (HMSN). The major contribution of Dyck and Lambert was to show that clinically identical CMT patients could be separated into two broad groups based on electrophysiologic and pathologic findings. The first (HMSN I, CMT 1) was characterized by severely reduced nerve conduction velocity and, on nerve biopsy, extensive and onion bulb changes. In the second (HMSN II, CMT 2) nerve conduction velocity was normal or only mildly reduced, and nerve biopsy showed loss of axons with little demyelination. These two patterns were consistent within families. Each of these two categories was shown to be genetically heterogeneous with both autosomal dominant and autosomal recessive inheritance patterns. An additional category with X-linked inheritance was later confirmed. It was shown that the Roussy-Lévy syndrome was a variant of CMT 1 and that it is totally distinct from Friedreich's ataxia.

This progressive splitting of Charcot-Marie-Tooth disease into multiple genetic entities was not an idle academic exercise. The identification of particular clinical syndromes with differing patterns of inheritance is vital for accurate genetic counseling, and it paved the way for the spectacular advances in the molecular genetics of CMT disease that have taken place in recent years. Hopefully, these will lead to an understanding of the underlying disease mechanisms and ultimately to effective treatment.

Charcot-Marie-Tooth disease is not rare, although estimates of its prevalence have varied considerably between different surveys, ranging from about 20 to over 40 per 100,000. The true figure is probably closer to the latter. Recognition of CMT disease is important. Fortunately, most patients with the disease remain ambulant and have an active and productive life. Proper orthopedic attention during childhood and adolescence can often prevent the development of serious foot and spinal deformity. In adult life, the provision of appropriate orthotic devices or corrective surgery may result in substantial functional benefit. Patients with severe sensory loss must be advised about foot care so that chronic foot ulceration or other foot problems do not result from inadvertent foot injury.

This book addresses the diagnosis and management of patients with CMT disease as it presents to the primary care physician. Our understanding of the disease has advanced very considerably in the past few years, and this knowledge can be translated into improved health care.

References

Dyck PJ, Lambert EH: Lower motor and primary sensory neuron diseases with peroneal muscular atrophy. I. Neurologic, genetic and electrophysiologic findings in hereditary polyneuropathies. *Arch Neurol*; 18:603 - 618, 1968.

Dyck PJ, Lambert EH: Lower motor and primary sensory neuron diseases with peroneal muscular atrophy. II. Neurologic, genetic and electrophysiologic findings in various neuronal degenerations. *Arch Neurol*; 18:619-625, 1968.

Gabreels-Festen A, Gabreels F: Hereditary demyelinating motor and sensory neuropathy. *Brain Pathol*; 3:135-146, 1993.

Hahn AF: Hereditary motor and sensory neuropathy: HMSN type II (neuronal type) and X-linked HMSN. *Brain Pathol*; 3:147-155, 1993.

Harding AE, Thomas PK: The clinical features of hereditary motor and sensory neuropathy, types I and II. *Brain*; 103:259-280, 1980.

Harding AE, Thomas PK: Autosomal recessive forms of hereditary motor and sensory neuropathy. *J Neurol Neurosurg Psychiatry*; 43:669 - 678, 1980.

Thomas PK, Harding AE: Inherited neuropathies: the interface between molecular genetics and pathology. *Brain Pathol*; 3:129 - 133, 1993.

THE CLINICAL FEATURES OF CHARCOT-MARIE-TOOTH DISORDERS

Carlos A. Garcia, M.D.

Professor, Departments of Neurology and Pathology
Louisiana State University School of Medicine in New Orleans.
Medical Director of the Muscular Dystrophy Clinics in Baton Rouge, Lafayette, and New Orleans, LA.
1542 Tulane Avenue, New Orleans, LA 70112-2822.

Key words: *Neuropathy, pes cavus, claw hands, steppage gait, slapping gait, hammer toes, hip dysplasia, scoliosis, kyphosis, essential tremor.*

Introduction

The clinical features of Charcot-Marie-Tooth (CMT) disorders are as heterogeneous as the genetic characteristics. Clinical signs and symptoms are frequently variable between different families and within the same family (1), including homozygous twins (2). Symptoms may range from severe weakness and wasting of leg and hand muscles along with bone deformities to mild symptoms or no symptoms at all. Asymptomatic patients may have a normal neurologic examination and may therefore have to be diagnosed by electrophysiologic studies and DNA analysis (3). Since the autosomal dominant form, CMT1A, is the most frequent form of this syndrome, a detailed clinical description of this variant will be given, and the other clinical forms will be compared to this type.

Reasons for Consultation

Only a few members of an affected family, usually the most affected ones, will consult a physician for their symptoms. The patients' most frequent complaints are loss of balance, gait disturbance, muscle weakness and foot deformities. Some patients are referred to the neurologist by orthopedic doctors or physiatrists because of abnormal nerve conduction studies. A few children are referred by their teachers because of clumsiness or idiopathic toe walking. Once the diagnosis is confirmed in one affected family member, other asymptomatic or symptomatic members may present for genetic counseling, for prescription of braces, or to seek disability compensation.

Age of Onset

The disease has an insidious onset over several years and such a slowly progressive course that some patients are unaware of their disease. The symptoms most frequently appear at the end of the first decade or early in the second decade and may be preceded by a slight delay in developmental milestones. The most frequent age of onset is between 12 and 19 years (4,5). Toe walking in childhood may be the first manifestation of the disease. Patients who are diagnosed in the second or third decade may reveal to the physician that they were always clumsy, never played sports in school, had difficulty running and could never keep up with childhood activities. Some older patients may have had surgical procedures to correct foot deformities in childhood prior to the diagnosis of the disease. The penetrance of the clinical phenotype may be low in the first decade but increases with age, although the penetrance of the electrophysiologic abnormality is essentially age independent. The chance of a patient showing first symptoms after the third decade decreases markedly.

Symptoms

A frequent complaint by patients is tripping over objects on the floor, which is due to a dropped foot that is caught by the object on the swing-through phase of the gait. Ankle sprains are also frequent and are due to weakness of dorsiflexion and eversion of the foot produced by weakness and atrophy of the anterior tibial muscles. Fractures of the ankles are not unusual. Older patients may complain of difficulty finding shoes to fit their small, high-arched feet and usually buy larger size shoes. Leg cramps are frequent and are worse after long walks. Hand cramps are reported by children after writing for long periods in school or by adults who do clerical work in an office. Lower back pain is most frequently seen in patients with uncorrected gait abnormalities and is probably due to the strain put on the paraspinous muscles during walking. Painful corns over the dorsal metatarsal heads of the toes and calluses over the lateral surface of the foot are frequent. However, pressure ulcers are rare. The most frequent complaint concerning hand involvement is difficulty buttoning, unbuttoning, using zippers, and manipulating small objects when using fine finger movements. Trying to pick up small objects with the fingers is difficult due to lack of approximation of the thumb with the other fingers. Also, the use of pliers, forks, spoons, and pencils is difficult. Opening screw cap tops on jars and turning doorknobs can also be difficult. Poor tolerance to cold weather is a frequent complaint, as is an excessive coolness in the legs. This complaint is often associated with trophic changes in the legs, such as loss of hair, edema, and discoloration of the skin of the legs. A decrease in skin and muscle temperature of 5°C to 10°C has been recorded (6), probably due to loss of muscle mass.

Occasional patients become severely disabled. Profound weakness of distal muscles makes activities of daily living extremely difficult. Weakness of proximal muscles of the legs may interfere with ambulation and patients may become wheelchair dependent. Even axial muscles may sometimes be involved, but significant impairment of respiratory function is extremely rare. There is a correlation between the severity of the conduction slowing at a young age and the ultimate development of a severe clinical deficit, so this more disabling outcome may be able to be predicted early.

General Physical Findings

The disease does not affect the life span, the intellectual functions, or the cardiovascular system. There are no systemic disorders associated with the disease, and associated neurologic findings are rare and will be mentioned below.

Gait

The patient should be asked to walk barefoot, since most patients walk better with the shoes on and even better with hightop shoes or boots. The gait abnormality is directly related to the severity of the leg muscle weakness and the skeletal deformity of the feet. Early in the course of the disease, the gait may look normal, but the physician may notice that the patient dorsiflexes the toes with each step. The earliest objective difficulty with gait is the inability of the patients to walk on their heels. As the disease progresses and the anterior tibial muscles get weaker, the foot drops with each step and the patient is forced to lift the knee and throw the foot and toes upward to avoid tripping over any object ("steppage gait"). The rapid descent of the foot to the floor produces the "slapping" noise that is heard when the patient walks ("slapping gait").

Weakness, Atrophy, and Muscle Stretch Reflexes

The muscle weakness in this disorder affects predominantly the distal muscles and is manifested by the gait disturbance and hand difficulties described above. The muscle weakness first begins in the intrinsic foot muscles and then ascends to affect the anterior tibial muscles. Then, the distal part of the gastrocnemius and the distal portion of the quadriceps muscles become weak. The leg muscles then become atrophic giving the appearance of "stork legs" or "inverted champagne bottles" in severely affected patients. However, a thick layer of subcutaneous fat, especially in women, may mask the leg muscle atrophy. The weakness and atrophy of the hand muscles usually occurs late in the course of the disease, but may not be related to the degree of leg weakness or atrophy and is not related to the age of the patient. The thumb usually rotates owing to weakness of the muscles of the thenar eminence, producing the simian hand. The fingers are semiflexed at all joints and there is interdigital wasting due to atrophy of the interossei muscles, which gives a guttering appearance to the dorsal surface of the hands. All these features produce the appearance of a claw hand. The muscle stretch reflexes may be normal in the early stages of the disease and in some asymptomatic affected patients with slowed nerve conduction velocities (NCV) (3). However, areflexia is seen in most patients first in the ankle, then in the patella, and finally in the upper limbs. The plantar response is invariably flexor.

Sensory and Autonomic Dysfunction

Sensory symptoms are rarely reported by the patients. However, decreased sensation in the legs in a stocking distribution is found in most patients. The upper limbs are usually not affected. In the legs, position sense is usually preserved but vibratory sense is decreased. Poor tolerance to cold weather and a decrease in the temperature of the legs as described above are frequent. Leg ulcers may occur in advanced cases in which the patient has foot deformities and are seen over the pressure points.

Enlarged Nerves

Enlargement of the superficial nerves may be seen or palpated in 20 - 25% of the patients (6). The enlargement of the nerves is not related to the age of the patient or the severity of the symptoms. Hypertrophy of the greater auricular nerve may be seen in the lateral surface of the neck in slender individuals. It is most frequently found in men and frequently may be seen or palpated more easily on one side than on the other. A thickened ulnar nerve may be palpated one or two inches above the ulnar groove. The enlarged peroneal nerve may be palpated behind the head of the fibula.

Bony Abnormalities

Pes cavus is variable, is usually not seen early in the disease, and seems to progress with age. However, it may be seen as early as in the first decade or may not be seen at all, even in some elderly patients. The heel cord is frequently tight. The pes cavus is characterized by a short foot with an abnormally high arch. This foot shape is produced by atrophy and weakness of intrinsic foot muscles and unopposed long toe flexors and extensors. There is also a plantar flexion and an internal rotation of the foot. In advanced cases, the toes become retracted in flexion, producing the "hammer toe" deformity. Pain is frequent, and the rare development of ulcers can occur in these patients. Pes planus occurs early in the disease and is seen in 10% of the patients. Scoliosis is usually mild with a very slow progression and is seen in only a few patients. However, juvenile kyphosis is more characteristic of the disease and may be quite severe in a few patients. Hip dysplasia in children with CMT is asymptomatic or minimally symptomatic and is only detected in early adolescence (7). Pain and a limp are the main manifestations, and the treatment is usually surgical.

Pulmonary Function

Restrictive lung disease is usually not a major problem in CMT patients. There is a low frequency of respiratory complications, and pulmonary function tests show only mild non-progressive impairment (8).

Essential Tremor

Tremor is not usually a complaint in patients with CMT, but, when specifically asked, 40% of the patients (9) respond positively. The tremor involves mainly the hands, and it may be present at any age but is usually first noted in the mid-30s. The tremor is not related to the severity of the symptoms of CMT and has all the clinical features of essential tremor. These features along with the high frequency of family history of tremor suggest that CMT and esssential tremor are either due to separate genes or are a variable expression of the same gene (9). What Roussy-Lévy described as a separate entity seems to be a combination of CMT and essential tremor.

Course and Outcome

CMT is a slowly progressive disease, and thus the severity of the symptoms is a time-dependent phenomenon. However, full clinical expression is completed by the third decade. In our population, which consists of predominantly autosomal dominant, CMT1A, the younger the patient at the onset of the symptoms the more severe the neurologic deficit. However, out of 250 patients, only two who are both in their 70s, are partially confined to a wheelchair. Most symptomatic patients continue to work in spite of their disability.

Clinical and Genetic Correlations

Most patients with CMT have similar clinical features. However, there are some forms of CMT that vary from the typical clinical pattern. The forms that vary usually also have a different inheritance pattern. To determine the type of CMT that the patient has, one must use a molecular genetic approach and a family pedigree and correlate these with the clinical features (see table). Some families with CMT were described before the new technologies were available, so molecular analysis needs to be applied to clarify the type of CMT that these families have (10). The clinical features of CMT1A, CMT1B, and CMT1C are identical. More than 70% of the autosomal dominant CMT1A patients show the DNA duplication in chromosome 17 p11.2-12 (11). Autosomal dominant CMT1A is also caused by point mutations in the PMP22 gene (12) which maps within the part of the chromosome that is duplicated in CMT1A. The autosomal dominant form of CMT1B, which is linked to chromosome 1, has been described as being slightly more severe clinically than CMT1A (6). CMT1C, is not linked to either chromosome 17 or chromosome 1 (13). An autosomal recessive form of CMT1 has been described (14) in which patients show more weakness and scoliosis and significantly lower median motor NCV. In the X-linked dominantly inherited type of CMT1 (CMT X1), there is no male to male transmission on the pedigrees and the males are more severely affected than the females (15). In the X-linked recessive form (CMT X2), female carriers transmit the disease to their sons.

There are several important differences between the CMT1 and the neuronal form, CMT2 (6, 16). In the autosomal dominant form of CMT2, the onset of symptoms is usually in the second decade and may be as late as in the seventh decade. The atrophy and weakness of the plantar flexor muscles is more severe and the weakness of the hand muscles is less severe than in type 1. In

Clinical and Genetic Correlations

	Age of onset	Hand weakness	Leg weakness	Enlarged Nerves	Muscle Stretch Reflexes	Motor NCV's	Wheelchair dependent	Observations
AD CMT1A (chromosome 17) with duplication of PMP22 with point mutation of PMP22	1st or 2nd decade	Affected late	Affected early	May be found	Absent	Prolonged	Rare and late	See text
AD CMT1B (chromosome 1) with point mutation in P_0	"	"	"	"	"	Prolonged	"	Slightly more severe clinically than CMT1A
AD CMT1C (No linkage to chromosome 1 or 17)	"	"	"	"	"	Prolonged	"	
AR CMT (No linkage found yet)	"	"	"	"	"	Intermediate	"	More weakness and scoliosis than CMT1
X-LINKED Dominant CMT X1	"	"	"	"	"	Prolonged	"	Males affected more severely than females
X LINKED Recessive CMT X2	1st or 2nd decade	Affected late	Affected early	May be found	Absent	Prolonged	Rare and late	Female carriers transmit the disease to males
AR CMT3 (Dejerine-Sottas)	Infancy	Severe	Severe	Present	Absent	Severely Prolonged	2nd or 3rd decade	Clinically similar to CMT1 homozygous
AD CMT2 (neuronal type)	2nd decade	Mild	Severe	Absent	Normal	Normal	Rare	Same phenotype as CMT1
AR CMT2 (neuronal type)	At birth or infancy	Severe	Severe	Absent	Normal	Normal	2nd decade	Severe clinical deficit

autosomal dominant CMT2 there is no enlargement of the nerves and the muscle stretch reflexes are normal. The sensory loss is less frequent, and the proprioception is the most frequently affected modality. Pes cavus deformity is less frequent, and the NCVs are normal. In the autosomal recessive form of CMT2, signs of the disease may be present at birth or may appear within the first three years of life. The age of walking is delayed, the hand involvement is more severe and begins earlier, and the progression of the disease is faster. Most patients become wheelchair dependent by the second decade. CMT3 or Dejerine-Sottas syndrome is a hypertrophic form of neuropathy that is usually autosomal recessive. The onset of symptoms occurs in infancy with motor developmental delay and abnormal gait. The patients are usually of short stature with full lips and coarse facial features. The progression of the disease is slow, but the patients are wheelchair dependent by the second or third decade. The nerves are hypertrophic and the NCVs are extremely slow. Homozygous patients with CMT1A have very similar features (17, 18, 19). In fact, in two families with a confirmed clinical diagnosis of Dejerine-Sottas syndrome, DNA analysis showed new point mutations on the PMP22 gene (20).

CMT Associated Features

Some families with CMT have been described that have features of other diseases and conditions, probably due to an independent gene(s). Spastic paraparesis, deafness, optic atrophy, Marfan-like appearance and absent eyebrows have been described in patients with CMT. Molecular analysis in these cases may clarify in the near future whether these clinical findings are due to the same or independent mutations (6).

Acknowledgments: I am grateful to the Muscular Dystrophy Association and to the patient service coordinators for their help in the clinics. I appreciate the cooperation of the predominantly Acadian-American CMT families of the Muscular Dystrophy clinics of Lafayette, Baton Rouge, and New Orleans, Louisiana. Finally, I greatly appreciate the editorial assistance of Ms. Alison Barbee and the help of Ms. Kathy Cantrell in the preparation of this manuscript.

References

1.Lupski JR, Garcia, CA, Parry GJ, et al.: Charcot-Marie-Tooth polyneuropathy syndrome: clinical, electrophysiologic and genetic aspects. In: *Current Neurology*, edited by Appel, S. Chicago: Mosby-Year Book, 1991, p 1-25.

2.Garcia CA, Malamut RI, Parry GJ, et al.: Clinical heterogeneity of HMSN1 in two pairs of identical twins. *Neurol* (supl) 40: 301, 1990.

3.Kaku D, Parry GJ, Malamut RI, et al.: Nerve conduction studies in Charcot-Marie-Tooth polyneuropathy associated with a segmental duplication of chromosome 17. In press. *Neurol.*

4.Bird TD, Ott J, Giblett ER, et al: Genetic linkage evidence for heterogeneity in Charcot-Marie-Tooth neuropathy (HMSN type 1). *Ann Neurol* 14: 679-684, 1983.

5.Bell J: On the peroneal type of progressive muscular atrophy. In: Fisher RH (Ed): *The treasure of human inheritance.* Vol IV, Part II. London, Cambridge University Press, 1935, pp 69-140.

6.Dyck PJ, Chance P, Lebo R, et al.: Hereditary Motor and Sensory Neuropathies. In: *Peripheral Neuropathy.* Edited by Dyck PJ, Thomas PK, Griffin J, Low PA and Poduslo JF. Philadelphia: WB Saunders Company. 1992, p 1094-1136.

7.Kumar SJ, Marks HG, Bown JR, et al: Hip dysplasia associated with Charcot-Marie-Tooth disease in the older child and adolescent. *J Ped Ortho* 5: 511-514, 1985.

8.Eichaker PQ, Spiro A, Sherman M, et al: Respiratory muscle dysfunction in Hereditary Motor Sensory Neuropathy, Type I. *Arch intern Med* 148: 1739-1740, 1988.

9.Cardoso FEC, Jankovic J: Hereditary motor-sensory neuropathy and movement disorders. *Muscle & Nerve* 16: 904-910, 1993

10.Lupski JR, Chancc P, Garcia CA: Inherited primary peripheral neuropathies: Molecular genetics and clinical implications. (in press).

11.Wise CA, Garcia CA, Davis S,N et al: Molecular analysis of unrelated Charcot-Marie-Tooth disease patients suggests a high frequency of the CMT1A duplication. *Am J Hum Genet* 53: 1993.

12.Rao BB, Garcia CA, Suter U, et al: Charcot-Marie-Tooth disease type 1A. Association with spontaneous point mutation in the PMP22 gene. *New Engl J Med* 329: 96-101, 1993.

13.Chance FF, Matsunami N, Lensch W, et al: Analysis of the DNA duplication 17p11.2 in Charcot-Marie-Tooth neuropathy type 1 pedigrees: additional evidence for a third autosomal CMT1 locus. *Neurol* 42: 2037-2041, 1992.

14.Gabreels-Festen AAWM, Gabreels FJM, Jennekens FGI, et al: Autosomal recessive form of hereditary motor and sensory neuropathy type I. *Neurol* 42: 1755-1761, 1992.

15.Ionasescu VV, Burns TL, Searby C, et al: X-linked dominant Charcot-Marie-Tooth neuropathy with 15 cases in a family genetic linkage studies. *Muscle & Nerve* 11: 1154-1156, 1988.

16.Harding AE, Thomas PK: The clinical features of hereditary motor and sensory neuropathy types I and II. *Brain* 103: 259-280, 1980.

17.Lupski JR, Montes de Oca Luna R, Slaugenhaupt S, et al: DNA duplication associated with Charcot-Marie-Tooth disease type 1A. *Cell* 66: 219-232, 1991.

18.Killian JM, Kloepfer HW. Homozygous expression of a dominant gene for Charcot-Marie-Tooth neuropathy. *Ann Neurol* 5: 515-522, 1979.

19. Sghirlanzoni A, Pareyson D, Balestrini MR, et al: HMSN III phenotype due to homozygous expression of a dominant HMSN II gene. *Neurol* 42: 2201-2203, 1992.

20. Rao BB, Dyck PJ, Marks HG, Chance PF, and Lupski JR: Dejerine-Sottas syndrome associated with point mutation in the PMP22 gene. *Nature Genetics* (in press).

ELECTRODIAGNOSTIC STUDIES IN CHARCOT-MARIE-TOOTH DISORDERS

Gareth J. Parry MD, FRACP

Professor of Neurology, University of Minnesota, Minneapolis
Medical Director of the Muscular Dystrophy Association Clinic

Key words: *CMT 1, CMT 2, electromyography, nerve conduction velocity*

The recording of nerve conduction is an integral part of the evaluation of any neuropathy; electromyography and nerve conduction studies are as important to neuropathies as electrocardiography is to heart disease. From a very early age, nerve conduction studies are abnormal in the autosomal dominant, hypertrophic form of Charcot-Marie-Tooth disease (CMT 1). Conduction slowing represents the most consistent phenotypic manifestation of this disease. Unfortunately they are less reliably abnormal in other forms of CMT, at least during the early phases of the disease, but they do become abnormal later. Electrodiagnostic studies may be used to establish the diagnosis of CMT neuropathy and are invaluable in screening family members. They are also useful for classifying the type of CMT neuropathy, in assessing the severity of the neuropathy for prognostic purposes, and in providing reproducible quantitative data for therapeutic or other experimental studies. These returns can be achieved cost-effectively with only modest discomfort to the patient.

What Are Electrodiagnostic Studies?

What is widely known in the medical and lay communities as "EMG" consists of recording bioelectrical signals from sensory and motor nerves and from muscle and using these to better understand the underlying pathology. The most important component of the electrodiagnostic study in CMT neuropathies is the recording of nerve conduction. To study nerve conduction, the nerves are activated with an electrical shock delivered through the skin to the underlying nerve. The electrical potential produced can be recorded directly from the nerve, some centimeters removed from the site of stimulation, or from the muscle which the nerve supplies. Direct recording from nerves is used to measure conduction in sensory nerves while motor conduction is measured by recording from muscles. Both stimulation of nerves and recording of nerve and muscle action potentials are usually done with surface electrodes; the only discomfort to the patient is from the electric shock. In normal individuals and in patients with certain types of neuropathy, this discomfort is negligible. In patients with CMT 1 the threshold for depolarization of the nerve is greatly elevated and a much stronger shock needs to be given, with an accompanying increase in the level of discomfort. However, most CMT patients, even young children, are remarkably tolerant of this part of the procedure as evidenced by the remarkable lack of difficulty I have experienced in getting patients to return for further studies. The true electromyography (EMG) part of the study entails recording electrical potentials from muscles using a needle electrode to pick up the activity. Multiple sites of several muscles need to be explored and each needle movement evokes some pain. In general, it is this part of the study which is less well tolerated but, fortunately, is less important in CMT neuropathies.

In nerve conduction studies, the parameters that can be measured are the amplitude of the sensory or motor response, which is evoked by the electrical stimulus, and the velocity of conduction along the nerve. These parameters are used to predict the underlying pathology of the nerve. The evoked motor response recorded from the muscle is called the compound muscle action potential (CMAP), and its amplitude is roughly proportional to the number of innervated muscle fibers in the muscle. The amplitude of the evoked sensory response recorded from the nerve, the sensory nerve action potential (SNAP), is proportional to the number of functioning sensory axons. Neuropathies in which the primary pathology is loss of axons, like CMT 2, therefore tend to have low amplitude responses, but conduction velocity is close to normal, as will be discussed later. Conduction velocity primarily reflects the state of myelination of nerve fibers; when there is demyelination and remyelination, as occurs in CMT1, conduction is very slow.

Abnormalities of the EMG reflect loss of motor axons. During the EMG, a needle electrode is inserted into a muscle and electrical activity is recorded at rest and during voluntary muscle contraction. At rest, normal muscles are electrically silent while denervated muscle fibers intermittently spontaneously depolarize, and this electrical potential can be recorded with an intramuscular needle electrode as a fibrillation. During voluntary contraction, the basic unit of the muscle, which consists of many muscle fibers innervated by a single motor axon, generates an electrical potential, the motor unit potential. Changes in the amplitude, duration, and configuration of the motor unit potential occur with chronic denervation and reinnervation. When motor axons degenerate, the denervated muscle fibers are quickly reinnervated by branches from adjacent surviving motor axons and individual motor unit potentials become larger and longer, and the configuration becomes more polyphasic. Because of this compensatory mechanism for preserving function, the loss of motor axons generally exceeds the loss of functioning muscle fibers in chronic neuropathies and other denervating disorders. In general, needle EMG is more sensitive than nerve conduction studies when evaluating neuropathies like CMT 2, in which the predominant pathology is axonal degeneration, but it is less well tolerated by most patients.

Electrodiagnostic Studies in CMT 1

- **Nerve Conduction Studies**

CMT 1, regardless of the manner of inheritance, has considerable phenotypic variability of its clinical manifestations; some patients are severely disabled while others are asymptomatic and are found only during routine family screening. However, all affected individuals, whether symptomatic or not, have slowed motor conduction velocity (MCV) from a very early age. In contrast, patients with CMT 2 usually conduct at rates which are close to normal. In one study, the mean MCV in the median nerve in the forearm in patients with CMT 1 was about 25 m/sec but, in some patients, it was as high as 42 m/sec (1); 45 m/sec was suggested as the upper acceptable limit of MCV in CMT 1. Other workers suggested the slightly lower figure of 38 m/sec as the value which separates CMT 1 from CMT 2 patients (2) and this has become the most widely used value. However, it is important to emphasize that this figure is only a guide and that occasional affected members of a CMT 1 pedigree will have conduction velocities slightly faster than 38 m/sec and CMT 2 patients may occasionally conduct more slowly, particularly when the disease is advanced. Although the clinical manifestations of CMT 1 are predominantly motor, sensory nerve conduction is also severely abnormal and sensory conduction velocity is similar to the MCV (3).

In CMT 1 patients, the MCV is normal at birth but it becomes abnormal very early in life, some time between four and six months of age (4,5). Until the age of about five years, the degree of slowing appears to worsen but it then remains stable for the remainder of life (6-8). It has therefore been suggested that five years of age is the optimal time to screen children for the disease, although it is obviously possible to diagnose the disease earlier.

The lack of change in conduction velocity during most of life suggests that the defect in myelination that characterizes CMT 1 is static after early childhood.

The degree of conduction slowing correlates poorly with the severity of the clinical deficit at any particular time during the course of the disease. During routine screening of families, some clinically normal children and adults are often found to have severe conduction slowing. Furthermore, as mentioned above, the inexorable progression of the disease is not paralleled by further slowing of conduction velocity. However, the severity of the conduction slowing may reflect the severity of the disease process, and patients with the most severe conduction slowing may ultimately develop the most severe neurologic deficit. Thus, Dyck and associates found that severe conduction slowing in early life was associated with more severe disease later in life (7). The clinical deficit in CMT1 results from the progressive axonal degeneration that is an inevitable consequence of the disease, rather than from the slow conduction velocity. As the neuropathy progresses, the amplitude of motor responses falls and evidence of denervation is seen with needle electromyography. There is a good correlation between the compound muscle action potential amplitude and the severity of the clinical deficit (6,7). Although the clinical manifestations of CMT 1 begin distally and progress proximally, conduction slowing, which reflects the defect in myelination, is strikingly uniform. The degree of conduction slowing is almost identical regardless of which nerve is studied or whether proximal or distal nerve conduction velocity is measured (4,9).

It was initially suggested that the degree of conduction slowing was almost identical in all affected members of a family. For example, Nielsen and Pilgaard (10) observed that conduction velocities were almost identical in two generations in four of their five families with CMT 1. However, their numbers were small and other studies have refuted this suggestion (1). We recently studied a group of 129 patients with CMT 1 and there were 4 families in whom we studied eight or more affected members. The range of conduction velocities in these families was large: 10-28 m/sec, 11-34 m/sec, 13-27 m/sec, and 20-40 m/sec (11). There was no reliable relationship between conduction velocity and age or apparent severity of disease as judged by clinical criteria. In one study of genetically confirmed identical twins, despite clinical heterogeneity, conduction velocities were identical (12).

- **Electromyography**

The needle EMG has little role to play in the diagnosis of CMT 1. Early in the course of the disease, EMG is normal since there is no axonal degeneration. As the disease progresses, axonal degeneration becomes inevitable and some evidence of denervation becomes apparent. The severity of the denervation is proportional to the severity of the clinical deficit, but there is little evidence that the EMG is any better at predicting future course than the clinical evaluation. Since the needle EMG is the least tolerated aspect of the electrodiagnostic studies, I use it sparingly in the evaluation of clinically involved CMT 1 patients and never in screening.

Electrodiagnostic Studies in CMT 2

- **Nerve conduction studies**

CMT 2 is characterized pathologically by degeneration of sensory and motor axons, rather than by demyelination and remyelination. Therefore, there is little slowing of conduction velocity; the velocity measured will essentially be that of conduction in the fastest of the surviving axons. In most patients with CMT 2 motor conduction velocity is greater than 40 m/sec, although slightly slower conduction may be seen in advanced disease (1,2). In asymptomatic individuals and those with mild neuropathy, the conduction velocity is almost always normal. Thus, using motor conduction velocity to screen families for covert disease has no utility. The amplitude of the compound muscle action potential (CMAP) is also preserved until the disease is advanced when there is severe loss of motor units. By the time the amplitude of the motor responses is reduced, there is always severe weakness and muscle atrophy. Early in the course of the disease, sensory nerve action potential amplitudes may be normal, but they are usually reduced; as the disease progresses, they disappear completely. The amplitude of the sensory nerve action potentials is, by and large, proportional to the clinical severity of the neuropathy so they are of limited usefulness in screening family members who have no clinical symptoms or signs of neuropathy.

- **Electromyography**

Needle EMG is somewhat more sensitive than the nerve conduction studies in unearthing covert abnormalities in CMT 2. However, the changes are mild and entirely nonspecific. There is seldom any fibrillation until the disease is advanced, since denervated muscle fibers are quickly reinnervated by collateral sprouting of nearby surviving axons. However, there are usually abnormalities of motor unit configuration and recruitment. Individual motor units tend to be of increased amplitude and duration and they are more likely to be polyphasic. These changes are initially confined to distal muscles since the most distal extent of the motor axons degenerate earliest; later, the changes are more widespread but remain distally accentuated. Unfortunately, essentially identical changes can be seen in any neuropathy in which there is axonal degeneration, as well as in radiculopathies.

Summary

Electrodiagnostic studies are always abnormal in CMT 1 and are invaluable in family screening, having essentially a 100% yield in detecting asymptomatic cases. They may also have some role in predicting the severity of future clinical deficits, when conduction slowing is severe at an early age. In CMT 2, the primary role of the electrodiagnostic studies is to distinguish among patients with the same CMT phenotype but who have different forms of the disease.

References

1. Dyck PJ, Lambert EH: Lower motor and primary sensory neuron diseases with peroneal muscular atrophy. I. Neurologic, genetic and electrophysiologic findings in hereditary polyneuropathies. *Arch Neurol*; 18:603-618, 1968.

2. Harding AE, Thomas PK: The clinical features of hereditary motor and sensory neuropathy types I and II. *Brain*;103:259-280, 1980.

3. Buchthal F, Behse F. Peroneal muscular atrophy (PMA) and related disorders. I. Clinical manifestations as related to biopsy findings, nerve conduction and electromyography. *Brain*; 100:41-66, 1977.

4. Berciano J, Combarros O, Calleja J, et al: The application of nerve conduction and clinical studies to genetic counseling in hereditary motor and sensory neuropathy type I. *Muscle Nerve*; 12:302-306, 1989.

5. Vanasse M, Dubowitz V: Dominantly inherited peroneal muscular atrophy (hereditary motor and sensory neuropathy type I) in infancy and childhood. *Muscle Nerve*; 4:26-30, 1981.

6. Gutmann L, Fakadej A, Riggs JE: Evolution of nerve conduction abnormalities in children with dominant hypertrophic neuropathy of the Charcot-Marie-Tooth type. *Muscle Nerve*; 6:515-519, 1983.

7. Dyck PJ, Karnes JL, Lambert EH: Longitudinal studies of neuropathic deficits and nerve conduction abnormalities in hereditary motor and sensory neuropathy type I. *Neurology* ; 39:1302-1308, 1989.

8. Roy EP, Gutmann L, Riggs JE: Longitudinal conduction studies in hereditary motor and sensory neuropathy type I. *Muscle Nerve*; 12:52-55 , 1989.

9. Kaku DA, Parry GJ, Malamut R, et al: Uniform slowing of conduction velocities in Charcot-Marie-Tooth polyneuropathy type I. *Neurology* 43:2664-2667, 1993.

10. Nielsen VK, Pilgaard S. On the pathogenesis of Charcot-Marie-Tooth disease: A study of the sensory and motor conduction velocity in the median nerve. *Acta Orthop Scand* 43:4-18, 1972.

11. Kaku DA, Parry GJ, Malamut R, et al: Nerve conduction studies in Charcot-Marie-Tooth polyneuropathy associated with a segmental duplication of chromosome 17. *Neurology* 43:1806-1808, 1993.

12. Garcia CA, Malamut R, Parry GJ, et al: Clinical heterogeneity in two pairs of identical twins. *Neurology* (in press).

PATHOLOGIC CHANGES IN CHARCOT-MARIE-TOOTH DISORDERS

John W. Griffin, M.D.

Professor of Neurology
Johns Hopkins University School of Medicine
Baltimore, Maryland

Key words: *axon, Schwann cells, myelin, demyelination, onion bulbs, Dejerine-Sottas, hypomyelinating neuropatihies*

This chapter will consider the organization of the normal nerve fiber and the variety of changes in that organization that occur in the different forms of Charcot-Marie-Tooth (CMT) disease. All of the cells in the body make use of the same classes of subcellular organelles, but in the cells of the nervous system these organelles are often highly specialized. For example, in most cells the cell nucleus with its deoxyribonucleic acid (DNA) can undergo division (mitosis) to produce daughter cells and renew the cell popoulation. Neurons and many of the supporting cells of the peripheral nervous system (PNS), the *Schwann cells*, normally do not divide after differentiation. Neurons *cannot* dedifferentiate and divide in any setting, but in disease the Schwann cells can proliferate vigorously.

The DNA of all cells also contains the genetic messages that instruct a specific type of ribonucleic acid (RNA), the messenger RNA (mRNA). This transcription of genetic instructions from DNA to RNA is followed by translation of the RNA into specific proteins. In many cell types, such as white blood cells or liver cells, the cell is relatively small and all elements of the cell are *near* the nucleus, a region called the *perikaryon*. In contrast, the major cell types of the nervous system are highly asymmetric. For example, the nerve cells that contribute to the peripheral nerves each extend a single long process, the *axon*, from the neuronal perikaryon, also called the *nerve cell body* (Figure 1). In the nerve fibers of the human sciatic nerve, this process may be over 3 feet in length and constitute a thousand-fold greater volume than the neuron's perikaryon. Yet virtually all of the protein-synthesizing machinery (the ribosomes and granular endoplasmic reticulum), as well as the nucleus, are located only in the nerve cell body. The axon is therefore necessarily dependent on the cell body for receipt of materials made there and conveyed to the axon by specialized forms of transport within the cells, the axonal transport systems.

Every axon in the peripheral nerve is surrounded or *ensheathed* by supportive Schwann cells. Around the larger axons, the Schwann cells elaborate a *myelin sheath* (Figure 2). Myelin is composed of the cell membrane of the Schwann cell, wrapped in a specialized lamellated fashion around and around the axon to produce a spiral of cell membrane many layers thick. In its biochemical make-up, the myelin sheath is somewhat different from the plasma membrane around other regions of the Schwann cell. It contains several substances that are specific or nearly specific for myelin, including the various myelin proteins.

The axon is covered by the myelin sheath along most of its extent, except for a short distance just outside the nerve cell body and a short distance from the nerve terminal. Each myelin sheath is produced by a single Schwann cell, and many of these sheaths are required to myelinate a long nerve fiber. In man, the longest myelin sheaths are 1.5-2 mm long (less than 1/10 of an inch). Between each adjacent myelin sheath is a very short distance of "uncovered" axon. These uncovered sites, which may be only 1 or 2 microns in length (1/25,000th of an inch), are called the *nodes*

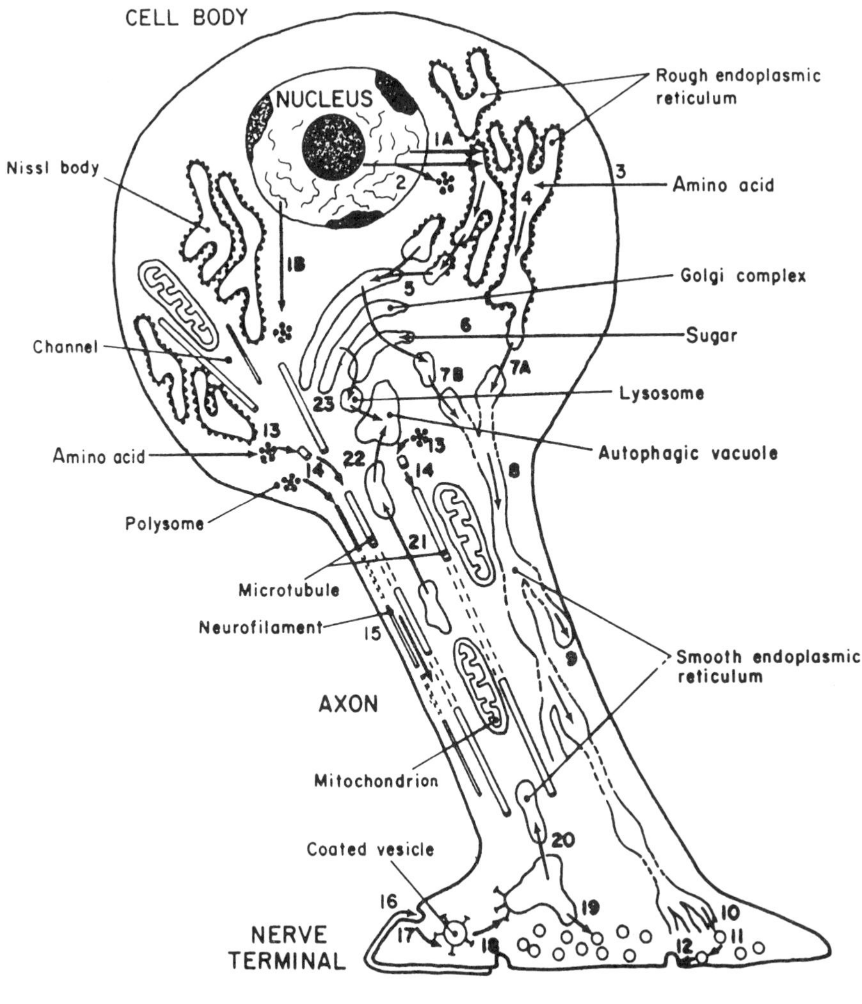

Figure 1. Schematic diagram of a neuron. Note that the nucleus and the protein-synthesizing organelles lie in the nerve cell body or perikaryon. The axon extends out from the perikaryon and lacks protein-synthesizing organelles. The myelin sheath is not shown.

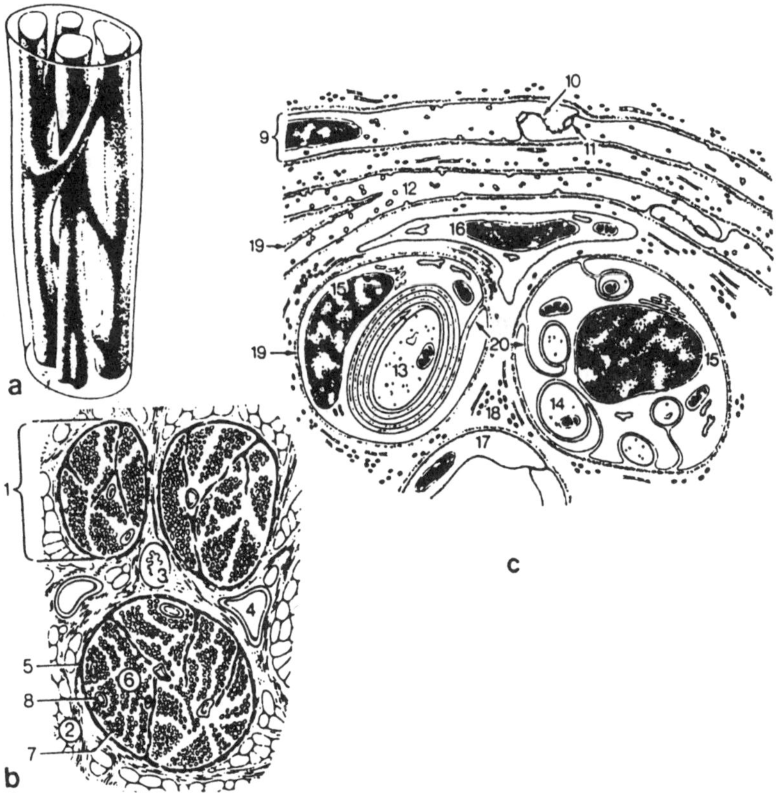

Figure 2. Organization of peripheral nerves.

A. Schematic diagram of a segment of nerve, demonstrating interlacing fascicles of nerve fibers.
B. Schematic diagram of a cross-section of nerve. 1. A single nerve fascicle. 2. Loose epineurial tissue. 3. An epineurial artery. 4. An epineurial vein. 5. Perineurium. 6. Endoneurial contents. 7. A bundle of myelinated fibers. 8. An endoneurial capillary.
C. Schematic diagram of a nerve fascicle as seen in the electron microscope. 9-12. Perineurial cells. 13. A large axon surrounded by a myelin sheath, together making up a myelinated nerve fiber. 14. A small axon in an unmyelinated nerve fiber. 15. Schwann cell nuclei. 16. Endoneurial fibroblasts. 17. Endothelial cell of an endoneurial capillary. 18. Endoneurial collagen. 19. Schwann cell basal lamina. 20. Mesaxons.

(Reprinted with permission from Mumenthaller M. and Schliack H., *Lasionin Peripherer Nerven* 4: Aufl., Thieme, Stuttgart, 1982.)

of Ranvier, after the 19th century scientist who first described them.

Normal function of a myelinated fiber depends on normal structure and function of both the axon and the myelin sheath. Peripheral nerve diseases can in general be divided into those that primarily affect the myelin sheath and those that primarily affect the axon. The inherited neuropathies, including the various forms of Charcot-Marie-Tooth disease, fit into this classification scheme (for review, see [1]). Thus, several of the types of Charcot-Marie-Tooth disorders discussed in this book represent abnormalities of the myelin-forming cells, and in some instances (the autosomal dominant forms CMT 1A and CMT 1B), the primary abnormalities are in specific myelin proteins (PMP-22 in CMT 1A [2-5], P_0 in CMT1B [6-9]). In the sex-linked recessive disorder, CMT X, the defect is in a protein, connexin 32 [10], which is found in cells throughout the body. To account for the abnormalities of myelin in CMT X, connexin-32 must play specific roles in the myelin-forming Schwann cells, but these roles are currently, poorly understood.

In all of these forms of CMT, the primary pathologic change is in myelin formation and maintenance. The myelin is too thin, the distances between nodes of Ranvier are too short, and the conduction of nerve impulses is too slow. Most importantly, at any time a small proportion of the myelin sheath is missing, a condition termed *demyelination*. These demyelinating forms will be considered in more detail.

In contrast, the other major class of CMT, CMT 2, has defects in maintenance of the axon. The axonal forms of Charcot-Marie-Tooth comprising CMT 2 are characterized by a loss of nerve fibers. The genetic defects underlying these disorders are not yet known. It seems likely that the defect or defects are in the neuron itself, but neurons depend on materials, including the various neuronal growth factors, made by target and supporting cells, so that a non-neuronal primary defect is possible.

Charcot-Marie-Tooth Type 1

CMT I in all its forms is dominated by evidence of myelin and Schwann cell abnormalities [11-15]. In the early and mid stages of these disorders, the number of nerve fibers is not substantially reduced, but many fibers are surrounded by myelin sheaths that are thinner than those in normal nerves. In addition, the fibers are more widely separated from each other as a result of several incomplete rings formed by extra (*supernumerary*) Schwann cells that surround each myelinated nerve fiber. As shown in Figures 3 and 4, these structures take up space, and as a consequence the entire nerve is enlarged or *hypertrophic*. These enlarged nerves can be felt or palpated in a number of sites (the ulnar nerve at the elbow, the peroneal nerve at the knee) and occasionally are visible, as in the greater auricular nerve in the neck. (See page 65, Figure 2, Chapter 6.)

These whorls of redundant Schwann cells are termed "onion bulbs," because of their obvious resemblance to a slice of onion, with its overlapping layers. Onion bulbs are seen not only in Charcot-Marie-Tooth disease, but also in some types of acquired demyelinating neuropathies. The precise conditions required for their development are not fully understood. They are often said to reflect demyelination and remyelination, but the story must be somewhat more complex. In experimental studies, after each episode of demyelination, the Schwann cell that has given up its myelin sheath divides and multiplies, as do the Schwann cells of neighboring unmyelinated nerve fibers [16]. These "daughter" Schwann cells typically surround demyelinated segments of the nerve fiber. Some of the daughter Schwann cells contact the axon

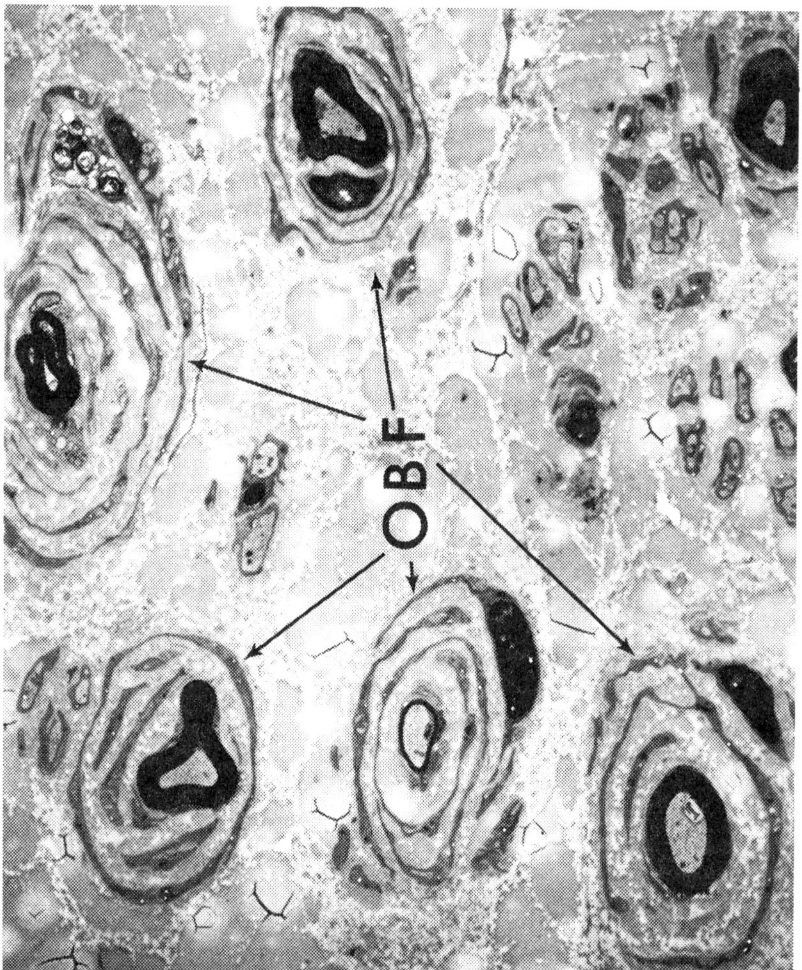

Figure 3
Hypertrophic changes in Charcot-Marie-Tooth disease 1A. The myelinated nerve fibers are surrounded by extra Schwann cell processes (examples identified by arrows). (OBF = onion bulb formations.)

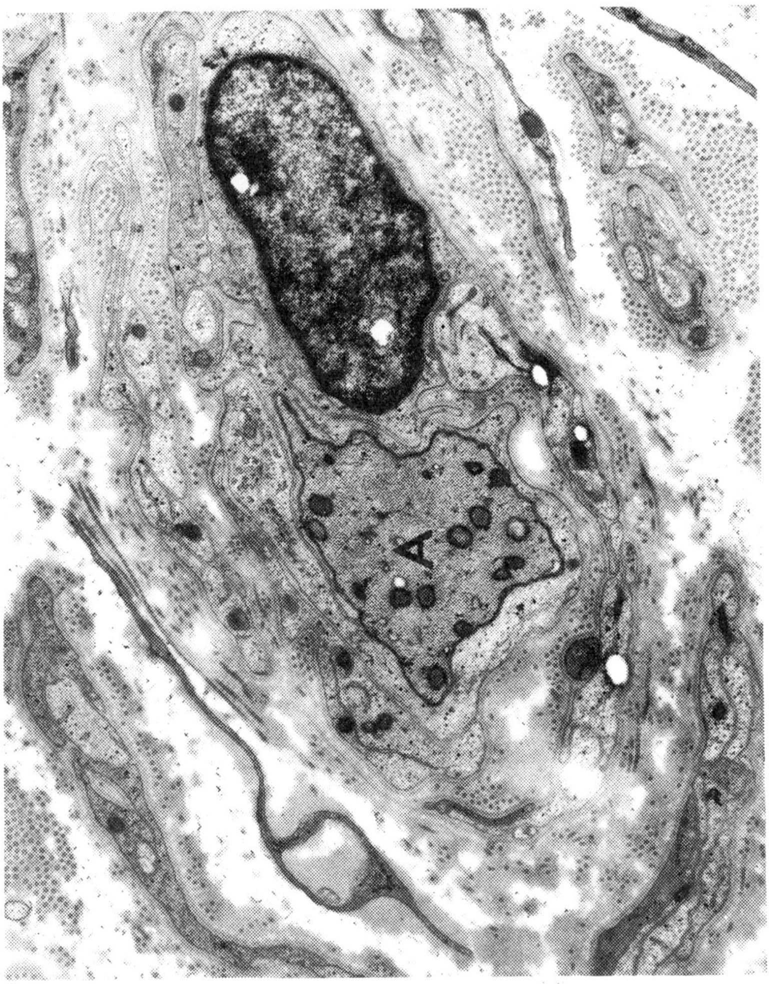

Figure 4
Electron micrograph of a single onion bulb in a patient with acquired demyelinating neuropathy.
(Reprinted with permission from Dyck, Thomas, Griffin, et al., *Peripheral Neuropathy*, W.B. Saunders, 1993.)

and ensheathe short segments. These successful daughter Schwann cells may then form short, thin myelin sheaths (*remyelination*). The daughter Schwann cells that are unsuccessful in reestablishing myelination typically become progressively smaller; their nuclei become darker in a fashion suggestive of less active cell synthesis; and they disappear, presumably as a result of cell death. Why, in CMT 1 and a few other settings, these daughter Schwann cells remain is uncertain, but their presence may reflect continuous proliferation or long survival of the daughter cells.

Nerves from CMT 1 usually have very little ongoing demyelination. True demyelination does occur in these disorders, but at any point in time only a few myelin sheaths are breaking down. Over time, however, this process cumulates and results in remyelination of most of the fibers. During the episodes of demyelination, the removal of myelin debris is carried out in part by special phagocytic cells (*macrophages*) that assist in the demyelinating process. Macrophage involvement is a non-specific response; macrophages appear to assist in removal of myelin debris in almost every type of peripheral nerve disease. Occasional degenerating fibers, in which the axon is breaking down, can be identified and, as the disease progresses, some overall loss of nerve fibers becomes the rule. In the most severe cases, a high proportion of the nerve fibers is lost, and the nerve contains mainly connective tissue, often with the organization of the old nerve fibers and their onion bulbs still detectable. This late loss of nerve fibers in diseases known to have the primary gene defect within the Schwann cell reflects the fact that survival of the axon depends on mutual interactions with the Schwann cell, so that disease in one produces abnormalities in the other.

Rarely the size of the onion bulbs and the resulting extent of nerve and nerve-root hypertrophy can, in themselves, cause symptoms. The enlarged nerve roots can be impacted in the spinal column or in the openings for the nerve roots from the spine (the *neural foramina*), causing nerve root or, in very rare cases, even spinal cord symptoms [17].

Dejerine-Sottas Disease

Dejerine-Sottas disease (CMT III or HMSN III) is distinguished from CMT 1 by a different pattern of inheritance (recessive), a different underlying gene abnormality (a mutation in the PMP-22 gene), and, in most instances, an earlier onset and often more severe neurologic dysfunction. The pathology is similar to that of CMT 1, but, in general, the myelin sheaths are thinner; more fibers without myelin sheaths are identified; and, the extent of nerve conduction slowing as measured physiologically is usually much more severe [13-15,18]. A frequent feature is the presence of "double basal lamina" in the onion bulbs [15,18]. Every Schwann cell forms a coating of extracellular matrix materials and collagen, its *basal lamina*. In Dejerine-Sottas, empty basal lamina, representing sites in which Schwann cells that formerly were arrayed within the basal lamina have disappeared, produce a collapsed serpentine sack. These structures are not specific, but, when numerous, are suggestive of Dejerine-Sottas disease.

Congenital Hypomyelinating Neuropathies

These are a large number of very rare disorders that present in early infancy. Children are born profoundly weak, often with difficulty swallowing, and frequently with tightly contractured joints (*arthrogryposis*), reflecting decreased movement of the fetus in the uterus. While there are many causes of arthrogryposis, the group of disorders under consideration here has a pathology characterized by extremely thin myelin or no myelin in the peripheral nerves. An example of such a nerve is shown in Figure 5 [19]. Pathologic studies suggested that the Schwann cells in this indi-

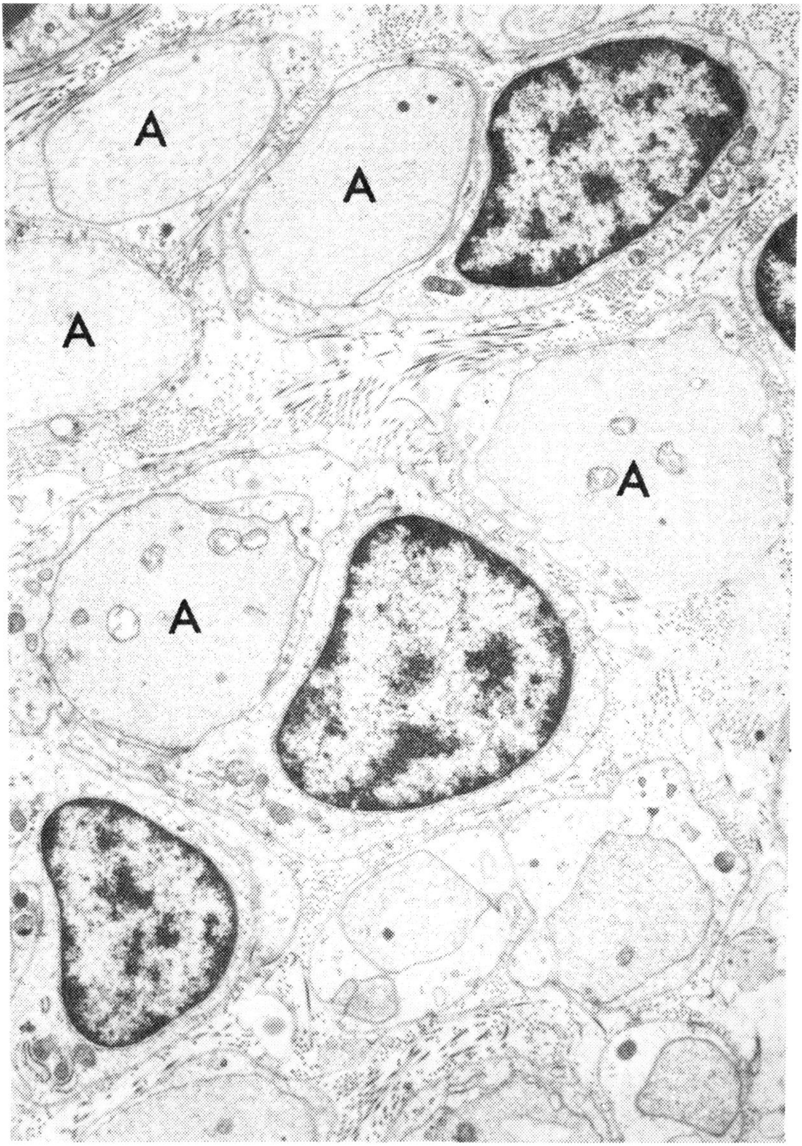

Fig. 5 A nerve from an infant with congenital amyelinating neuropathy and arthrogryposis. The axons are ensheathed by Schwann cells but no myelin has formed.

vidual's nerves were not able to grow longitudinally or radially in normal fashion.

Charcot-Marie-Tooth II

The clinical picture, electrophysiology, and pathology of CMT 2 all reflect a form of slowly evolving axonal degeneration that affects the long, large fibers of the peripheral nervous system initially. Over time, the process progresses to involve more proximal regions. Neither the gene defects nor the defects in the neurons have yet been discovered.

References

1 Chance PF, Pleasure D. Charcot-Marie-Tooth syndrome [Review]. *Arch Neurol* 1993;50:1180-1184

2 Valentijn LJ, Bolhuis PA, Zorn I, Hoogendijk JE, van den Bosch N, Hensels GW, Stanton VP,Jr., Housman DE, Fischbeck KH, Ross DA, et al. . The peripheral myelin gene PMP-22/GAS-3 is duplicated in Charcot-Marie-Tooth disease type 1A. *Nat Gen* 1992;1:166-170

3 Lupski JR, Wise CA, Kuwano A, Pentao L, Parke JT, Glaze DG, Ledbetter DH, Greenberg F, Patel PI. Gene dosage is a mechanism for Charcot-Marie-Tooth disease type 1A. *Nat Gen* 1992;1:29-33

4 Roa BB, Garcia CA, Pentao L, Killian JM, Trask BJ, Suter U, Snipes GJ, Ortiz-Lopez R, Shooter EM, Patel PI, et al. Evidence for a recessive PMP22 point mutation in Charcot-Marie-Tooth disease type 1A. *Nat Gen* 1993;5:189-194

5 Timmerman V, Nelis E, Van Hul W, Nieuwenhuijsen BW, Chen KL, Wang S, Ben Othman K, Cullen B, Leach RJ, Hanemann CO, et al. The peripheral myelin protein PMP-22 is contained within the Charcot-Marie-Tooth disease type 1A duplication [published erratum appears in Nat Genet 1992;2:84]. *Nat Gen* 1992;1:171-175

6 Kulkens T, Bolhuis PA, Wolterman RA, Kemp S, te Nijenhuis S, Valentijn JE, et al. Deletion of the serine 34 codon from the major peripheral myelin protein P_0 gene in Charcot-Marie-Tooth disease type 1B. *Nat Gen* ;5:35-39, 1993.

7 Hayasaka K, Himoro M, Sato W, Takada G, Uyemura K, Shimizu N, Bird TD, Conneally PM, Chance PF. Charcot-Marie-Tooth neuropathy type 1B is associated with mutations of the myelin P_0 gene. *Nat Gen ;* 5:31-34, 1993.

8 Himoro M, Yoshikawa H, Matsui T, Mitsui Y, Takahashi M, Kaido M, Nishimura T, Sawaishi Y, Takada G, Hayasaka K. New mutation of the myelin P_0 gene in a pedigree of Charcot-Marie-Tooth neuropathy 1. *Biochem Mol Biol Int*; 31:169-173, 1993.

9 Su Y, Brooks DG, Li L, Lepercq J, Trofatter JA, Ravetch JV, Lebo RV. Myelin protein zero gene mutated in Charcot-Marie-Tooth type 1B patients. *Proc Natl Acad Sci USA* 1993;90:10856-10860

10 Bergoffen J, Scherer SS, Wang S, Scott MO, Bone LJ, Paul DL, Chen K, Lensch MW, Chance PF, Fischbeck KH. Connexin mutations in X-linked Charcot-Marie-Tooth disease. *Science* 1993;262:2039-2042

11 Hughes JT, Brownell B. Pathology of peroneal muscular atrophy (Charcot-Marie-Tooth disease.) *J Neurol Neurosurg Psychiatry* 1972;35:648-657

12 Dyck PJ, Lais AC, Ohta M, Bastron JA, Okazaki H, Groover RV. Chronic inflammatory polyradiculoneuropathy. *Mayo Clin Proc* 1975;50:621-637

13 Dyck PJ, Lambert EH. Lower motor and primary sensory neuron diseases with peroneal muscular atrophy: I. Neurologic, genetic, and electrophysiological findings in hereditary polyneuropathies. *Arch Neurol* 1968;18:603-618

14 Dyck PJ, Lambert EH. Lower motor and primary sensory neuron diseases with peroneal muscular atrophy: II. Neurologic, genetic, and electrophysiological findings in various neuronal degenerations. *Arch Neurol* 1968;18:619-625

15 Ouvrier RA, McLeod JG, Conchin TE. The hypertrophic forms of hereditary motor and sensory neuropathy. A study of hypertrophic Charcot-Marie-Tooth Disease. (HMSN Type 1) and Dejerine-Sottas Disease (HMSN Type 3) in childhood. *Brain*; 110:121-148, 1987.

16 Griffin JW, Drucker N, Gold BG, Rosenfeld J, Benzaquen M, Charnes LR, Fahnestock KE, Stocks EA. Schwann cell proliferation and migration during paranodal demyelination. *J Neurosci*; 7:682-699, 1987.

17 Rosen SA, Wang H, Cornblath DR, Uematsu S, Hurko O. Compression syndromes due to hypertrophic nerve roots in hereditary motor sensory neuropathy type I. *Neurology*; 39:1173-1177, 1989.

18 Gabreels-Festen AA, Gabreels FJ, Jennekens FG, Joosten EM, Janssen-van Kempen TW. Autosomal recessive form of hereditary motor and sensory neuropathy type 1. *Neurology*; 42:1755-1761, 1992.

19 Charnas L, Trapp BD, Griffin JW. Congenital absence of peripheral myelin. *Neurology*; 38:966-974, 1988.

GENETICS OF CHARCOT-MARIE-TOOTH DISORDERS

Jeffrey M. Vance, M.D., Ph.D.

Key words: *Charcot-Marie-Tooth disease, Charcot-Marie-Tooth type 1, Charcot-Marie-Tooth type 2, Charcot-Marie-Tooth type 4, X-linked Charcot-Marie-Tooth, genetic heterogeneity, peripheral neuropathy, Hereditary Motor and Sensory Neuropathy, PMP-22, P_0, Connexin 32*

Introduction

Charcot-Marie-Tooth disease (CMT) is not only one of the most commonly inherited diseases in man, but also is now one of the classic examples of *genetic heterogeneity*. Genetic heterogeneity is defined as the phenomenon of mutations in different genes (usually on different chromosomes) independently producing the identical phenotype, or clinical appearance. Not only is CMT caused by many different genes (Figure 1), but these can be inherited in different patterns (Table 1). Therefore, to accurately provide information to a CMT family one must know not only the type of CMT (CMT1 or CMT2), but also the inheritance pattern of CMT in the family. Currently, (1995) over nine different gene mutations can cause the same CMT phenotype following both autosomal dominant or X-linked inheritance patterns. In addition, CMT can be inherited as an autosomal recessive disorder (CMT 4). While CMT4 has a similar clinical presentation to the more common autosomal dominant and X-linked forms, its earlier onset and greater severity often differentiates it from these types.

Review of Inheritance Patterns and Terms

There are two basic ways to approach the variability found in CMT:

Table 1

TYPE		LOCATION	DEFECT
Autosomal Dominant			
CMT 1			
	CMT 1A	17p11.2	microduplication or point mutation
	CMT 1B	1q22.3	Defect on P_0
	CMT 1C	unknown	
CMT 2			
	CMT 2A	1p36	unknown
	CMT 2B - ?	unknown	other type(s) not yet identified
X-linked CMT		Xq13	Connexin 32
Autosomal Recessive			
CMT4			
	CMT4A	8q13	unknown
	CMT4B-?	unknown	
	CMT4C-?	unknown	

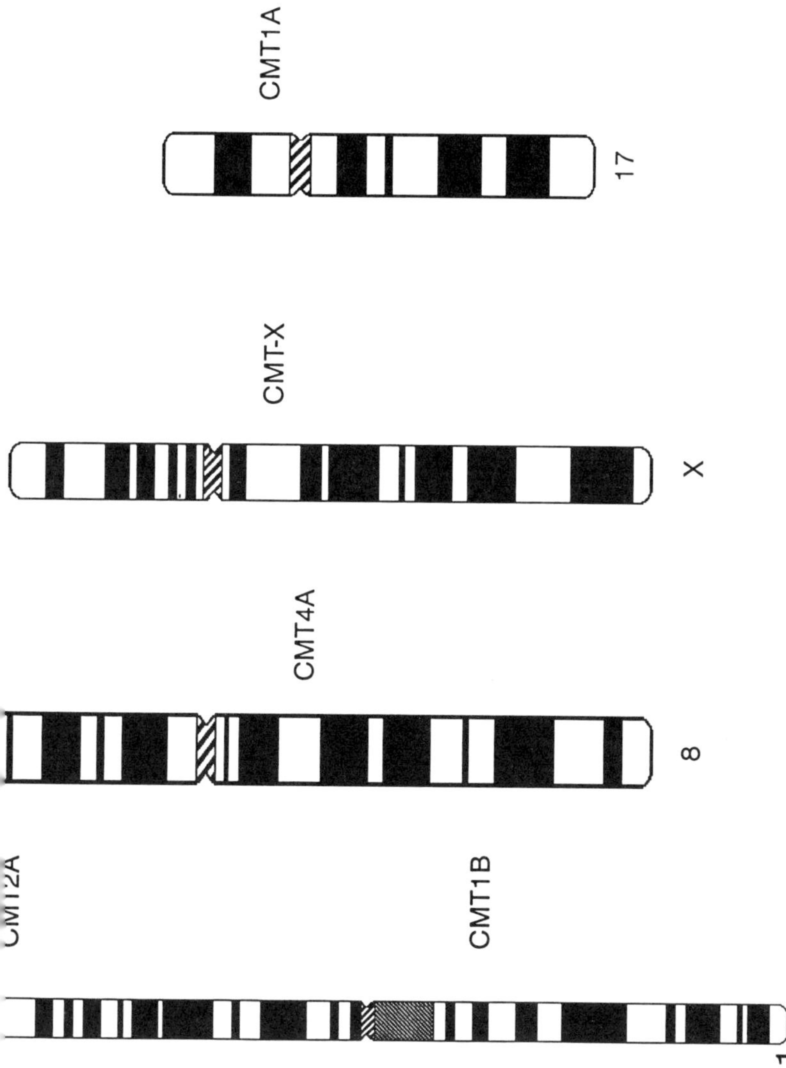

Figure 1. Present known chromosomal locations of genes causing the CMT phenotype.

1) to differentiate the different forms by pathologic or electrophysiologic findings, as in the divisions of CMT1 and CMT2, or

2) by the different inheritance patterns observed in the disorder.

In this chapter we will approach CMT through the different patterns of inheritance and mutations that make up its genetic heterogeneity.

Before discussing CMT directly, a few general principles should be reviewed. Genes are grouped together like "beads on a string" into chromosomes. While genes contain the blueprints for each protein, it is individual chromosomes that we inherit from our parents. Each cell contains 23 pairs of chromosomes, with chromosome 1 being the largest and chromosome 22 the smallest. All chromosomes come in pairs, so that each individual cell has two copies of every gene. The twenty-third pair of chromosomes is the X and Y chromosomes. The presence of a Y (XY pair) chromosome determines the child will be a male, while the absence of a Y (XX pair), which is replaced by a second X chromosome, produces a female child.

A genetic disease caused by a single gene defect can be inherited in one of five different patterns: autosomal dominant, autosomal recessive, X-linked recessive, X-linked dominant and mitochondrial. We will ignore mitochondrial inheritance in this discussion as it does not pertain to CMT. The term *autosomal* refers to any gene that does not lie on the X or Y chromosome pair. Each separate copy of a gene on a chromosome is called an *allele*. Alleles of a pair may be identical (homozygous) or have small nucleic acid base sequence differences between them, which usually does not affect function. If this variation occurs in greater than one percent of the population it is termed a *polymorphism*. Individuals with 2 different alleles in their chromosome pair are termed heterozygotes.

The exact pattern of inheritance (dominant or recessive) that a disease follows depends on the normal function of the defective protein that leads to the disease and the type of genetic mutation that is passed through a family. If only one copy (allele) of the disease gene in the gene pair is enough to cause the disease, the disease gene is *dominant* to the normal allele. This is an autosomal dominant disease. However, if the disease is produced only when both alleles of the gene pair are the abnormal disease gene, then the disease is *recessive* to the normal allele. This would be a recessive disease. In a recessive disease, individuals who have only one copy (or allele) of the disease gene and one copy of the normal gene are therefore clinically normal, but are disease gene *carriers.*

Examples of autosomal dominant and autosomal recessive inheritance patterns are shown in Figure 2. Compare those to Figure 3, where an X-linked pattern of inheritance is shown. In *X-linked inheritance* the gene causing the disease is located on the X chromosome. Therefore, in males, who have only one X chromosome, any abnormal X chromosome gene is the only gene they will have and therefore they will always demonstrate the disease. However, females may or may not demonstrate an X-linked disease. If the disease is *X-linked dominant,* carrier females will have the disease (like autosomal dominant), but usually their phenotype will not be as severe as affected carrier males, because they still have one normal gene. An *X-linked recessive disease* affects only those males carrying the abnormal gene. Females with one disease gene will be clinically normal, but are gene carriers. Female carriers of the *X-linked CMT* gene may or may not have symptoms, but if present their symptoms usually are not as severe as those of affected males. Therefore, the phenotype of X-linked CMT lies somewhere between the X-linked recessive and X-linked dominant phenotypes (1).

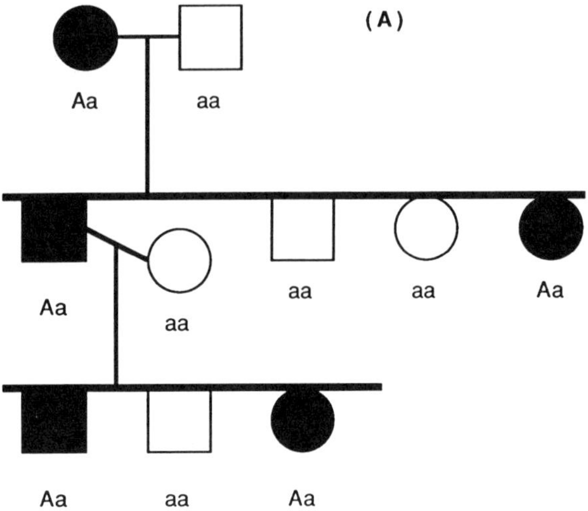

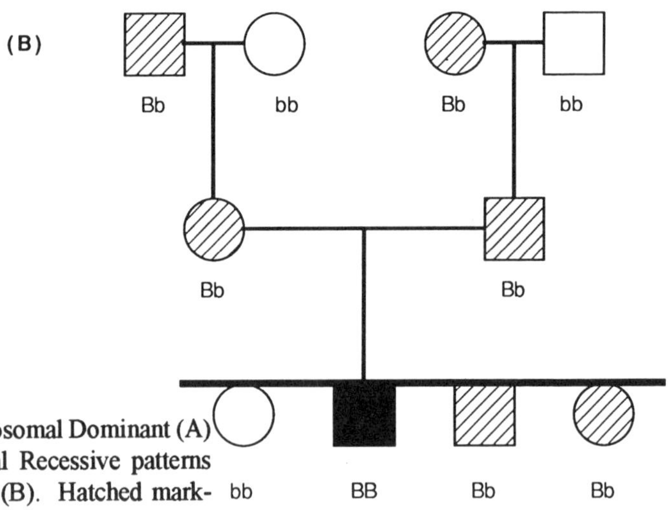

Figure 2. Autosomal Dominant (A) and Autosomal Recessive patterns of inheritance (B). Hatched markings represent carriers; darkened symbols are affected individuals. Square = male, circle = female.

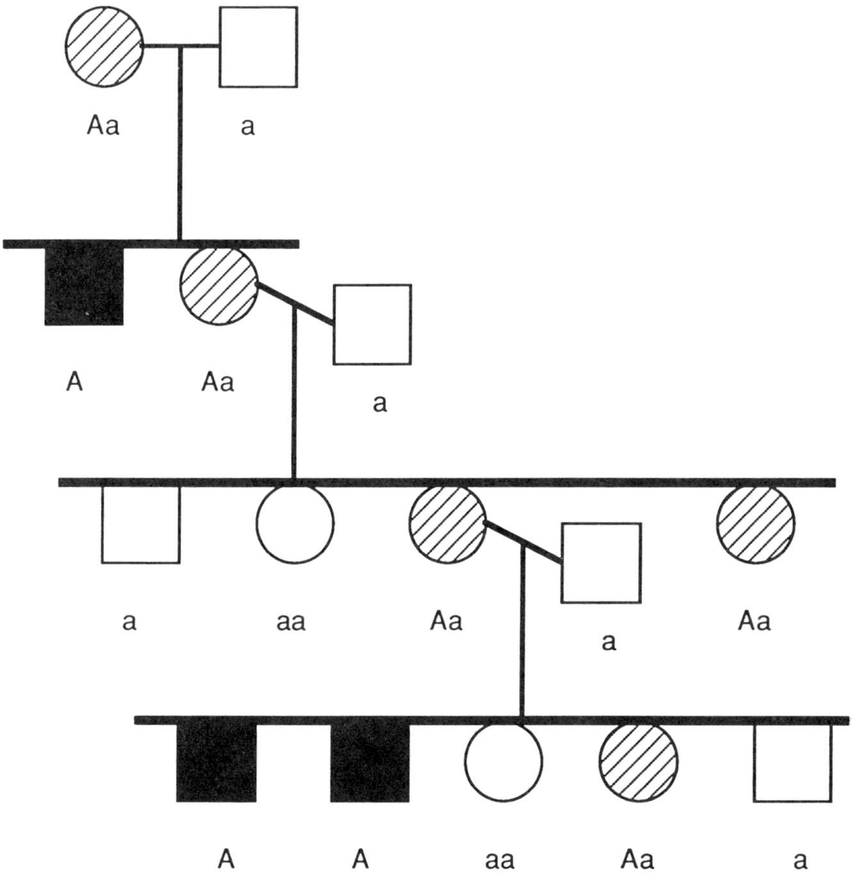

Figure 3. An example of X-linked inheritance. Females are carriers (hatched) while males inheriting the large "A" allele are affected.

Autosomal Dominant CMT

The majority of families with CMT in North America and Europe follow an autosomal dominant inheritance pattern. Both CMT1 and CMT2 include families that inherit the disease in this manner (2).

Individuals with autosomal dominant CMT have a 50% or one-half risk of passing the gene to their children. The sex of the child or the parent does not matter in this case. This risk of one-half arises because each parent provides to each child only one of the two chromosomes that make up the parental pair. The selection of which chromosome to give in the pair is usually random. The important thing to remember is that this risk (one in two) is for each child, as "chance has no memory." For example, even if the first nine children from a parent affected with autosomal dominant CMT did not inherit the CMT gene, the risk for the tenth child is still one in two.

- **CMT 1**

At least three different gene defects are known that cause CMT type 1 (demyelinating CMT, with slow nerve conductions): types A, B, and C. The gene defects for the vast majority (95%) of autosomal dominant CMT type 1 are located on chromosome 17p11.2 (3) (CMT1A). Within this classification of CMT1A two different mutations are known to exist: the majority (probably 60-80%, although this number is not yet known) have a large area of the chromosome duplicated (1.5 million base pairs, a microduplication), which is unique to CMT1A and thought to lead to the disease (Figure 4) (4,5). The other CMT1A families do not have a microduplication. Instead they have an abnormal base pair substitution in the gene that produces the myelin protein PMP-22 (6). This gene (PMP-22) is known to lie within the microduplica-

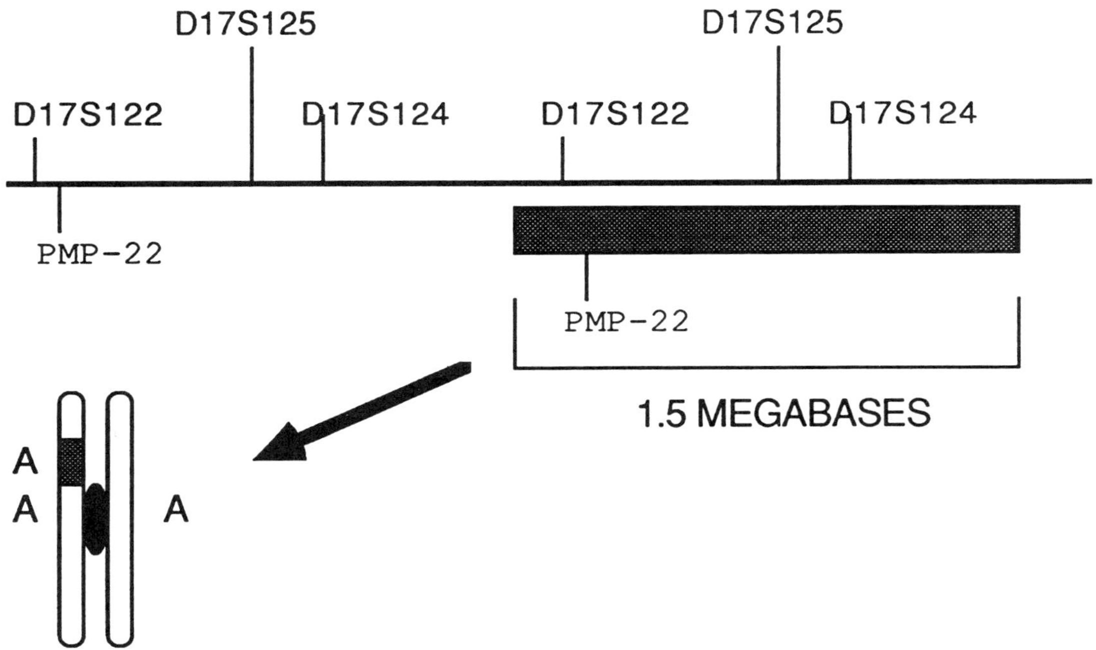

Figure 4. CMT1 A duplication. The duplication is linear on the chromosome and produces 3 copies of genes (A) contained within the duplication.

tion as well (7,8). Therefore, it is presumed, although not yet completely proven, that both the duplication of the PMP-22 gene (producing three copies of the gene instead of the normal two) and a single base mutation in PMP-22 can lead to CMT1A.

CMT1B is located on chromosome 1q22 (9) (Figure 1). The disorder has been recently shown to be caused by a genetic defect in another myelin protein, P_0 (10-12). Only a handful of families have been found to have this form of the disease. How these abnormalities produce CMT is currently under investigation. Finally, there are a few additional families that do not have their gene defects at either the CMT1A or CMT1B locations (13). The chromosomal location of these rare families is not known, but these families are currently termed CMT1C.

- **CMT 2**

CMT2 has been estimated to represent approximately one third of the CMT phenotype (14). This is surely an underestimate, as, in many cases seen by physicians, the family history is not appreciated and they are classified as nonspecific axonal neuropathies. Most families with CMT2 follow an autosomal dominant inheritance pattern. Recently our laboratory has demonstrated that at least two or more different genes cause this type of CMT (15). Currently, estimates suggest that 40-50% of CMT2 families have their genetic defect on chromosome 1, near the top, in region 1p36 (Figure 1). This type of CMT2 is now known as CMT2A. This is a different region of the chromosome from CMT1B. Currently the genetic defect is not known in CMT2A, nor the location of the other genes that lead to CMT2.

X-Linked CMT

Almost all X-linked CMT is classified as type 1. It is often difficult to tell if a family has the X-linked form of CMT1 or the autosomal dominant form. However, *if an affected male has an affected boy, then the disease cannot be X-linked.* (That is because to have a boy child, the father has to provide the Y chromosome instead of the X, and therefore, by definition, cannot transmit an X-linked disease to his male offspring).All the female offspring of an affected male with X-linked CMT will be carriers for CMT. One half of the offspring (regardless of the sex of the child) of a female carrier of X-linked CMT will inherit the gene.

The gene for X-linked CMT had been closely linked to the androgen receptor located in Xq13. Recently, work by a series of laboratories has identified the defect in X-linked CMT as Connexin 32, a gap junction protein (16). Because gap junction proteins had not been previously known to function in normal peripheral nerve, this finding should provide new insight into the neurophysiology of the peripheral nerve.

Autosomal Recessive CMT

This form of CMT has been described in Europe and North America for over 50 years. However, because of its inheritance pattern, it is much less common in these regions than in North Africa and South America, where the incidence of inbreeding is higher. Usually both parents of an affected child are clinically normal "disease carriers". They have a 25% recurrence risk to have an affected child.

Recently our laboratory has demonstrated that the gene for one of these forms, CMT4A, is located on chromosome 8q13 (17) (Figure 1). Most likely at least two other genes can cause CMT4 (types B and C), although the location of these types is not known. The genetic defect in CMT4A is not yet known.

Genetic Diagnosis

Genetic counseling in CMT is much more complex than it was just a few years ago. As initially discussed, the counselor needs to determine the type (CMT1 or CMT2) of CMT and then the inheritance pattern in the family of interest. Presently, only *direct* molecular testing is commercially available for CMT1A. However, testing for both CMT1B (P_0) and X-linked CMT (Connexin 32) should be available in the near future.

However, when direct testing is not available, a second form of genetic testing for carrier or affected gene status employs *linkage analysis*. This is a technique that is applied to a wide range of different genetic disorders. A detailed discussion is beyond this chapter, but an example is shown in Figure 5. Blood samples are taken from several family members to determine the alleles of normal DNA *polymorphisms* that lie very close on the chromosome to the disease (CMT) gene. The test can be used to try to determine which of these "linked" polymorphic alleles is inherited with the disease as it travels through the family. Then, if an individual inherits those alleles located on the "CMT chromosome," they will have a high probability of also inheriting the CMT gene. Currently this technique is not available for CMT on a regular basis but may well be in the future. Its drawbacks include the requirement that several members of a family must be available to participate, often excluding small families, and its results can never be 100% accurate.

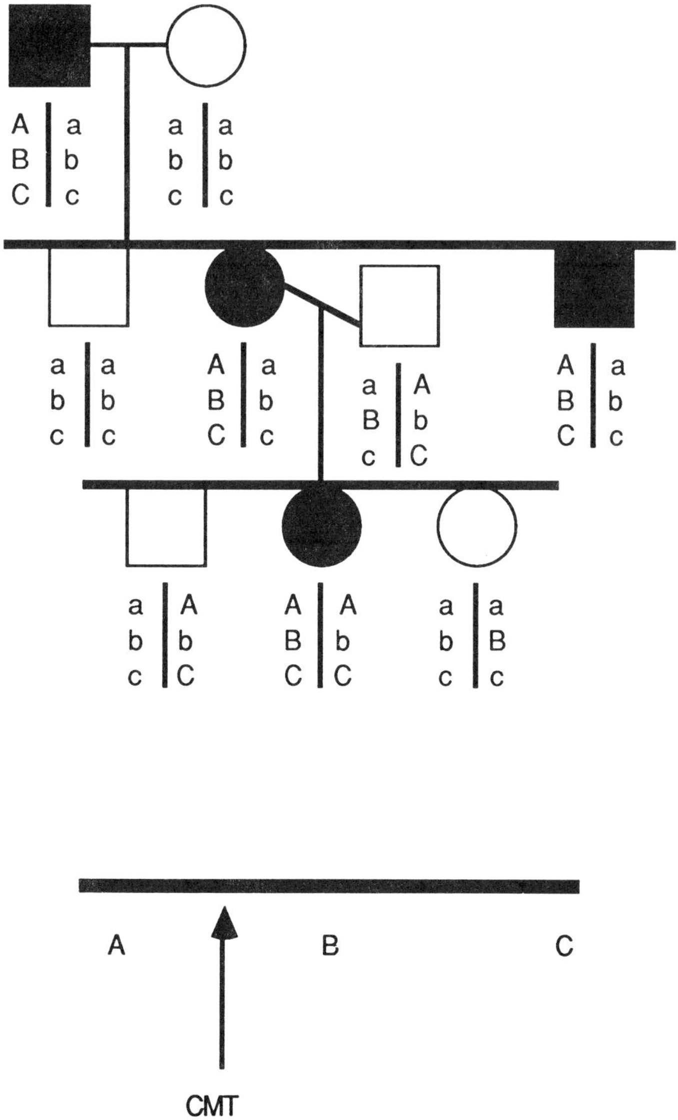

Figure 5. An example of genetic linkage. (A,a,), (B,b), and (C,c) are three markers surrounding the CMT locus. The CMT locus lies somewhere between markers A and B. In this case the gene defect for the CMT phenotype in this family is not known. However, one could predict the probability of inheriting the CMT gene based on whether any at-risk individual in the family inherits the chromosome containing the A, B, and C alleles (the "CMT chromosome") or the normal chromosome containing the a, b, and c alleles.

Summary

The CMT phenotype not only continues to be one of the most commonly inherited diseases of mankind, but certainly one of the most genetically complex. The limited sensitivity of past clinical, nerve conduction and electromyographic examinations in defining these diseases is now quickly being replaced by definitive genetic classifications. Therefore, it is no longer sufficient to refer to these patients as having CMT disease, implying a single entity. Rather, these disorders would be better termed the CMT phenotype, comprised of an increasingly complex set of different genetic diseases. The continuing elucidation of this phenotype will not only provide insight into these disorders, but also a window to the mechanisms of the normal peripheral nerve.

References

1. Rozear, M. P., M. A. Pericak-Vance, K. Fischbeck, J. M. Stajich, P. C. Gaskell Jr., D. A. Krendel, D. G. Graham, D. V. Dawson, and A. D. Roses. 1987. Hereditary motor and sensory neuropathy, X-linked: A half century follow-up. *Neurol.* 37:1460-1465.

2. Vance, J. M. 1991. Hereditary motor and sensory neuropathies. *J. Med. Genet.* 28:1-5.

3. Vance, J. M., G. A. Nicholson, L. H. Yamaoka, J. Stajich, C. S. Stewart, M. C. Speer, W. -Y. Hung, A. D. Roses, D. Barker, and M. A. Pericak-Vance. 1989. Linkage of Charcot-Marie-Tooth Neuropathy Type 1a to Chromosome 17. *Exp. Neurol.* 104:186-189.

4. Lupski, J. R., R. M. Montes de Oca-Luna, S. Slaugenhaupt, L. Pentao, V. Guzzetta, B. J. Trask, O. Saucedo-Cardenas, D. F. Barker, J. M. Killian, C. A. Garcia, A. Chakravarti, and P. I. Patel. 1991. DNA duplication associated with Charcot-Marie-Tooth Disease type lA. *Cell* 66:219-232.

5. Raeymaekers, P., V. Timmerman, E. Nelis, P. De Jonghe, J. E. Hoogendijk, F. Baas, D. F. Barker, J. J. Martin, M. De Visser, P. A. Bolhuis, and C. Van Broeckhoven. 1991. Duplication in chromosome 17p11.2 in Charcot-Marie-Tooth neuropathy type 1a (CMT1a). *Neuromuscular Disorders* 1:93-97.

6. Valentijn, L. J., F. Baas, R. A. Wolterman, J. E. Hoogendijk, N. van den Bosch, I. Zorn, A. A. W. M. Gabreels-Festen, M. De Visser, and P. A. Bolhuis. 1992. Identical point mutations of PMP-22 in Trembler-J mouse and Charcot-Marie-Tooth disease type 1A. *Nature Genetics* 2:288-291.

7. Timmerman, V., E. Nelis, W. Van Hul, B. W. Nieuwenhuijsen, K. L. Chen, S. Wang, K. Ben Othmane, B. Cullen, R. J. Leach, C. O. Hanemann, P. De Jonghe, P. Raeymaekers, G-J. B. van Ommen, J-J. Martin, H. W. Muller, J. M. Vance, K. H. Fischbeck, and C. Van Broeckhoven. 1992. The peripheral myelin protein gene PMP-22 is contained within the Charcot-Marie-Tooth disease type 1A duplication. *Nature Genetics* 1:171-175.

8. Patel, P. I., B. B. Roa, A. A. Welcher, R. Schoener-Scott, B. J. Trask, L. Pentao, G. J. Snipes, C. A. Garcia, U. Francke, E. M. Shooter, J. R. Lupski, and U. Suter. 1992. The gene for the peripheral myelin protein PMP-22 is

a candidate for Charcot-Marie-Tooth disease type 1A. *Nature Genetics* 1:159-165.

9. Lebo, R. V., P. J. Dyck, P. F. Chance, M. C. King, E. Lynch, M. Redila-Flores, J. S. Golbus, L. A. Anderson, C. C. Christian, R. R. Flandermeyer, M. van der Ploeg, J. Weigant, O. Hurko, D. Cornblath, D. R. Johns, T. D. Bird, Y. W. Kan, B. D. Bruce, L. G. Jackson, E. Epstein, G. Peltz, K. Moore, M. M. Shull, J. B. Lingrel, P. Green, S. Gendler, N. Latov, R. E. Lovelace, D. Dickoff, R. Blostein, S. A. Schonberg, L. S. Jenkens, V. Ionasescu, L. Gutman, G. Nicholson, L. Kadasi, V. Ferak, W. M. Rowler, J. Trofatter, and P. M. Conneally. 1989. Charcot-Marie-Tooth locus in FC-gamma-RII gene region. *Am. J. Hum. Genet.* 45:A148.(Abstr.)

10. Hayasaka, K., A. Ohnishi, G. Takada, Y. Fukushima, and Y. Murai. 1993. Mutation of the myelin P_0 gene in Charcot-Marie-Tooth neuropathy type 1. *Biochem. Biophys. Res. Commun.* 194:1317-1322.

11. Hayasaka, K., M. Himoro, W. Sato, G. Takada, K. Uyemura, N. Shimizu, T. D. Bird, P. M. Conneally, and P. F. Chance. 1993. Charcot-Marie-Tooth neuropathy type 1B is associated with mutations of the myelin P_0 gene. *Nature Genetics* 5:31-34.

12. Kulkens, T., P. A. Bolhuis, R. A. Wolterman, S. Kemp, S. te Nijenhuis, L. J. Valentijn, G. W. Hensels, F. G. I. Jennekens, M. De Visser, J. E. Hoogendijk, and F. Baas. 1993. Deletion of the serine 34 codon from the major peripheral myelin protein P_0 gene in Charcot-Marie-Tooth disease type 1B. *Nature Genetics* 5:35-39.

13. Chance, P. F., T. D. Bird, P. O'Connell, H. Lipe, J. M. Lalouel, and M. Leppert. 1990. Genetic linkage and heterogeneity in type I Charcot-Marie-Tooth disease (hereditary motor and sensory neuropathy type I). *Am. J. Hum. Genet.* 47:915-925.

14. Harding, A. E. and P. K. Thomas. 1980. The clinical features of hereditary motor and sensory neuropathy types I and II. *Brain* 103:259-280.

15. Ben Othmane, K., L. T. Middleton, L. J. Loprest, K. M. Wilkinson, F. Lennon, M. P. Rozear, J. M. Stajich, P. C. Gaskell, A. D. Roses, M. A. Pericak-Vance, and J. M. Vance. 1993. Localization of a gene (CMT2A) for autosomal dominant Charcot-Marie-Tooth disease type 2 to chromosome 1p and evidence of genetic heterogeneity. *Genomics* 17:370-375.

16. Bergoffen, J., K. Chen, B. W. Nieuwenhuijsen, S. Cochrane, N. Fairweather, A. Monaco, N. Haites, and K. H. Fischbeck. 1993. Localization of X-linked Charcot-Marie-Tooth Disease to Xq13.1. *Am. J. Hum. Genet.* 53:977.(Abstr.)

17. Ben Othmane, K., F. Hentati, F. Lennon, P. H. Denton, D. Loeb, C. Ben Hamida, S. Blel, A. D. Roses, M. Ben Hamida, M. A. Pericak-Vance, and J. M. Vance. 1993. Linkage of a locus (CMT4A) for autosomal recessive Charcot-Marie-Tooth disease to chromosome 8q. *Human Molecular Gentics* 2:1625-1628.

CHARCOT-MARIE-TOOTH DISORDERS IN CHILDREN

Harold Marks, M.D.

Chief, Division of Neurology
A.I. duPont Institute

Key words: *CMT 1 & 2, pes cavus, scoliosis, hip dysplasia, sensory loss, autonomic neuropathy, treatment*

Charcot-Marie-Tooth Disease (CMT) is a genetically heterogeneous disorder which clinically can be subdivided into two major types: the hypertrophic form of CMT (CMT type 1) and the axonal form of CMT (CMT type 2) . Both types usually have onset in childhood.

CMT is the most common inherited peripheral neuropathy. Prevalence of this disorder is most likely underestimated since, especially in children, this condition is often underdiagnosed or misdiagnosed. In adults, prevalence is reported to be 1 in 2500 (1), and in children ages 2-15 years approximately 19 per 100,000 (2).

Clinical Presentation

In most patients with CMT initial symptoms develop in the first 2 decades of life. About 5% of children with CMT are reported by parents to have abnormally shaped feet at birth, and, by their second birthday, about a third are symptomatic (3). In patients with CMT1 approximately 60% will have onset of symptoms in the first decade and 80% before the age of 20 years. In patients with CMT2 approximately 25% will have onset of symptoms in the first decade and a little more than half before the age of 20 years (4,5).

Most children with CMT are brought to the physician by their parents because of a foot deformity or abnormal gait. Young children may present with toe walking and adolescents with frequent ankle sprains. Other reasons for evaluation include family history, pain in ankles or feet, leg cramps, scoliosis, and hip dysplasia.

Clinical Findings

The clinical findings in children with CMT1 and CMT2 are similar, with findings usually being more severe in CMT1. They can be subdivided into orthopedic and neurologic problems.

Orthopedic complications are common (see Table I) and parents may take their children to an orthopedic surgeon before a neurologist. Almost all children with CMT have a foot deformity. The most common of these deformities is pes cavus (78%), which is often associated with a varus heel and claw toes (Figure 1). Flat feet are seen in about 11% of children. Other orthopedic problems include scoliosis and hip dysplasia. Scoliosis is reported in 10-16% of children (6,7,8), is usually mild, and infrequently requires bracing or surgery. An uncommon and often unrecognized orthopedic complication is hip dysplasia. It usually is asymptomatic or minimally symptomatic and may go undetected until early adolescence (9).

Neurologic findings include distal weakness and atrophy. The lower extremities are involved earlier and to a greater degree than the upper extremities. In the lower extremities, the anterior tibial muscle (foot dorsiflexors), the peroneal muscles (foot everters), and the extensor hallucis longus (long toe extensor) are clinically

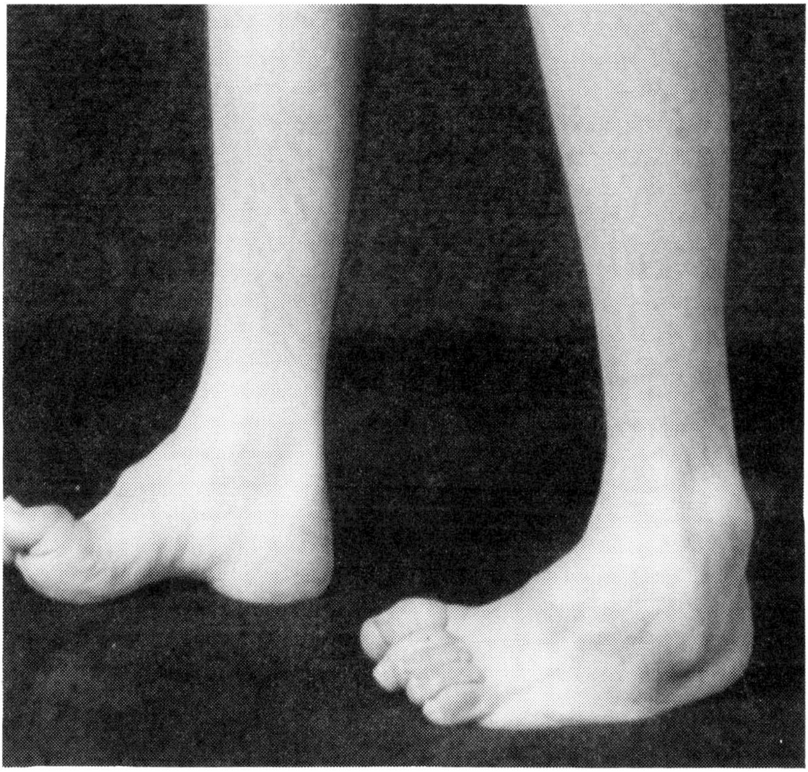

Figure 1. Fourteen-year-old boy with CMT1. Note cavus foot and claw toes on right foot and heel varus on left foot.

weak. Although lower extremity weakness and cavus deformities are usually symmetric, occasionally asymmetric involvement is seen. As the disease progresses, distal atrophy develops and patients may develop the classic "stork-leg" appearance. In the upper extremities, weakness involves the intrinsic muscles of the hand with the abductor digiti minimi (abductor of the small finger) being involved early. As weakness progresses, the patient may develop more proximal weakness and clawing deformities of the hand. This is uncommon in childhood.

Mild sensory loss is also seen. There is reduced pin-prick and temperature sensation in a stocking and glove distribution. Vibration sense is also reduced but abnormal proprioception is rare.

Although CMT1 is usually more severe than CMT2, there is a large clinical overlap and deep tendon reflexes (DTRs) may help to differentiate between the two types. In CMT1, there is usually total areflexia (55%) or markedly depressed DTRs, whereas in CMT2 reflex loss is usually limited to the ankles. Another clinical finding which may also help differentiate CMT1 from CMT2 is nerve hypertrophy, which is seen in approximately 50% of CMT1 and never in CMT2. The best nerve to evaluate is the greater auricular nerve in the neck (Figure 2).

In children, tremor is seen more commonly in CMT1 (25%) than in CMT2 (7%). The tremor is usually mild and similar to that seen with essential tremor having both a positional and volitional component.

Other neurologic abnormalities that have been rarely associated with CMT in children include sensory neural deafness (10,11), optic atrophy (12), and nemaline myopathy (13). The last was felt to have been inherited independently from CMT. Although sweating may be mildly impaired and patients commonly complain of cold hands and feet, other abnormalities of autonomic function are minimal in CMT1 and CMT2 (14).

Prognosis

CMT is a slowly progressive disorder, even in children with very early onset (7). CMT1 is generally more severe than CMT2. In Hagberg & Westerberg's (2) series, 20% of children with CMT were noted to have normal or near normal gait; 70% had an abnormal gait and difficulty running, and 10% were said to be

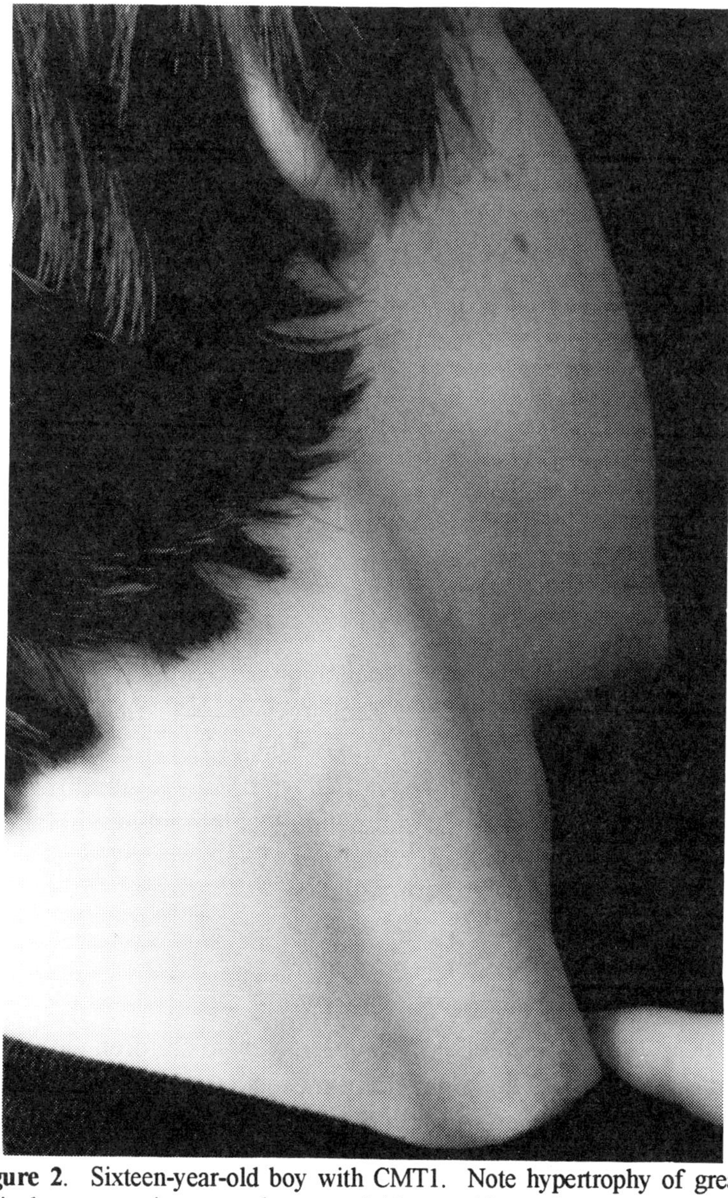

Figure 2. Sixteen-year-old boy with CMT1. Note hypertrophy of greater auricular nerve as it crosses the sternocleidomastoid muscle.

dependent on a walking aid or a wheelchair. None of the children with CMT2 were in the last category. My experience with CMT1 differs, and I would estimate that less than 5% of children with CMT1 need assistive ambulation or are wheelchair bound.

Treatment

Treatment is symptomatic. It includes bracing, physical therapy, orthopedic surgery and educational and psychological support. These have been discussed in other chapters, but I would like to make the following comments in regard to children. Most children do well with a home program of physical therapy and bracing. When the disease is first diagnosed, the child and family should be instructed in simple heel cord stretching exercises. It is impor-

Orthopedic Abnormalities in Children with CMT

	TOTAL	CMT1	CMT2
Number of cases	64	36	28
Cavus feet	50 (78%)	29 (80%)	21 (75%)
Flat feet	7 (11%)	3 (8%)	4 (14%)
Scoliosis	18 (28%)	10 (28%)	8 (28%)
Hip dysplasia	6 (9%)	5 (14%)	1 (4%)
Toe Walking	8 (13%)	5 (14%)	3 (11%)

tant that the heel cord not tighten since once it becomes tight it usually needs surgical release. In older children and adolescents referral to a physical therapist to instruct the family on a home program of stretching is appropriate. I encourage children to remain as active as possible. I ask that they not participate in contact sports but limitation in physical activities is something that needs to be determined with consideration given to the child's disability,the child's and family's wishes, and the family understanding of the risk of injury. I know an adult with CMT who runs marathons and another who skis every winter. I have seen children who have a great desire to play contact sports such as football, and with good conditioning, excel in their sport without suffering injuries.

It should be noted that older children, especially teenagers, do not wish to be different from peers and often resist the use of braces or going to physical therapy. In these children, instead of referring them to a physical therapy program, I will send them to a sports medicine program (an accepted alternative) and suggest that instead of wearing braces they wear high-topped tennis shoes or a supramalleolar orthosis (a foot orthosis with lateral hindfoot support). The latter may improve gait and give enough ankle support so that they can remain active and not frequently fall or twist an ankle.

Bibliography

1 Skre, H.: Genetic and clinical aspects of Charcot-Marie-Tooth disease. *Clin Genetics,* 6:98-118, 1974.

2 Hagberg, B., Westerberg, B.: Hereditary motor and sensory neuropathies in Swedish children. *Acta Paediatric Scand* 72:379-383, 1983.

3 Hagberg, B., Westerberg, B.: The nosology of genetic peripheral neuropathies in Swedish children. *Develop. Med. Child Neurol.* 25:3-18, 1983.

4 Harding, A.E.,Thomas, P.K.: The Clinical Features of Hereditary Motor and Sensory Neuropathy Types I and II. *Brain,* 103:259-280, 1980.

5 Bouche, P., Gherardi, R., Cathala, H.P., *et al.*: Peroneal Muscular Atrophy. *J Neurol Sci,* 61:389-399, 1983.

6 Hensinger, R.N., MacEwen, G.D.: Spinal deformity associated with heritable neurological conditions: Spinal Muscular Atrophy, Friedreich's Ataxia, Familial Dysautonomia, and Charcot-Marie-Tooth Disease. *J Bone and Joint Surg,* 58-A:1:13-24, 1976.

7 Vanasse, M., Dubowitz, V.: Dominantly inherited Peroneal Muscular Atrophy (Hereditary Motor and Sensory Neuropathy Type I) in infancy and childhood. *Muscle Nerve* 4:26-30, 1981.

8 Westerberg, B., Hagne, I., Sellden, U.: Hereditary motor and sensory neuropathies in Swedish children. *Acta Paediatr Scand* 72:685-693, 1983.

9 Kumar, S.J., Marks, H.G., Bowen, J.R., *et al*: Hip dysplasia associated with Charcot-Marie-Tooth disease in the older child and adolescent. *J Pediatric Orthopedics,* 5:511-514, 1985.

10 Bosenberg, R.N., Chutorian, A.: Familial Opticoacoustic Nerve Degeneration and Polyneuropathy. *Neurology,* 17:9:827-832, 1967.

11 Hamiel, O.P., Raas-Rothschild, A., Upadhyaya, M., *et al*: Hereditary Motor-sensory Neuropathy (Charcot-Marie-Tooth disease) with nerve deafness: A new variant. *J Pediatrics,* 123:3:431-434.

12 McLeod, J.G., Low, P.A., Morgan, J.A.: Charcot-Marie-Tooth disease with leber optic atrophy. *Neurology*, 28:179-184, 1978.

13 Danon, M.J., Sarpel, G., Manaligod, J.R.: Nemaline rod myopathy and Charcot-Marie-Tooth disease. *Arch Neurol*, 37:123-125, 1980.

14 McLeod, J.G.: Autonomic dysfunction in peripheral nerve disease. *J Clin Neurophysiol*, 10:1:51-60, 1993

15 Gutmann, L., Fakade, A., Riggs, J.E.: Evolution of nerve conduction abnormalities in children with dominant hypertrophic neuropathy of the Charcot-Marie-Tooth type. *Muscle Nerve*, 6:515-519, 1983.

16 Lupski, J.: An inherited DNA rearrangement and gene dosage effect are responsible for the most common autosomal dominant peripheral neuropathy: Charcot-Marie-Tooth disease type 1A. *Clin Research*, 40:4:645-652, 1992

17 Kaku, D.A., Parry, G.J., Malamut, R., *et al*: Nerve conduction studies in Charcot-Marie-Tooth polyneuropathy associated with a segmental duplication of chromosome 17. *Neurology*, 43:1806-1808, 1993.

18 Hoogendijk, J.E., Hensels, G.W., Gabreels-Festen, A.A., et al: De-novo mutation in Hereditary Motor and Sensory Neuropathy type I. *Lancet*, 339:1081-1082, 1992.

ORTHOPEDIC CONSIDERATIONS FOR CHARCOT-MARIE-TOOTH DISORDERS

John D. Hsu, M.D., C.M., F.A.C. S.

Chief of Orthopedics, Chairman, Department of Surgery
Co-Director, Muscular Dystrophy Association Clinics
Rancho Los Amigos Medical Center, Downy, California, USA
Clinical Professor, Department of Orthopedics
University of Southern California, School of Medicine.

Key words: *contractures, kyphoscoliosis, sprains, callosities, ankle, thumb, arthrodesis*

The orthopedic deformities seen in Charcot-Marie-Tooth (CMT) disorders are mainly in the hands and feet. However, other areas of the body can also be involved. Mild scoliosis, kyphosis, and kyphoscoliosis are seen. The hips may also be affected.

The deformities associated with the muscle weakness in patients with CMT generally develop slowly. An affected person can be asymptomatic and may have no complaints for a long period of time. If other members of the family are affected, the weakness may be noticed earlier. Frequently, the deformities cause minor problems and are viewed as annoyances. Personal adaptations, substitutions, or change of activity or lifestyle may have occurred before a complaint is brought to the attention of a physician.

Ankle and Foot

Weakness of the ankles, involuntary turning in and turning out of the ankle, tiredness in foot, mild aches around the ankle and foot, loss of balance, difficulty in walking with the eyes closed, frequent ankle sprains, and the formation of calluses on the outside of the foot can occur early. The manifestations of CMT neuropathies can start when a patient notices persistent turning in of the foot or trouble walking on uneven ground. This requires no treatment. The development of a high arch, callouses with toe deformities, hammer toes, and sensory changes occur later in the more advanced state (1). When the person with a high arch stands and walks, the callosities that develop on the plantar surface of the feet at the metatarsal heads may cause pain. Figure 1 shows the feet of a 17-year-old male and demonstrates some of these features. If there is turning of the foot, walking occurs on the outside of the foot and skin changes can occur with thickening of the skin and calluses generally at the 5th metatarsal head.

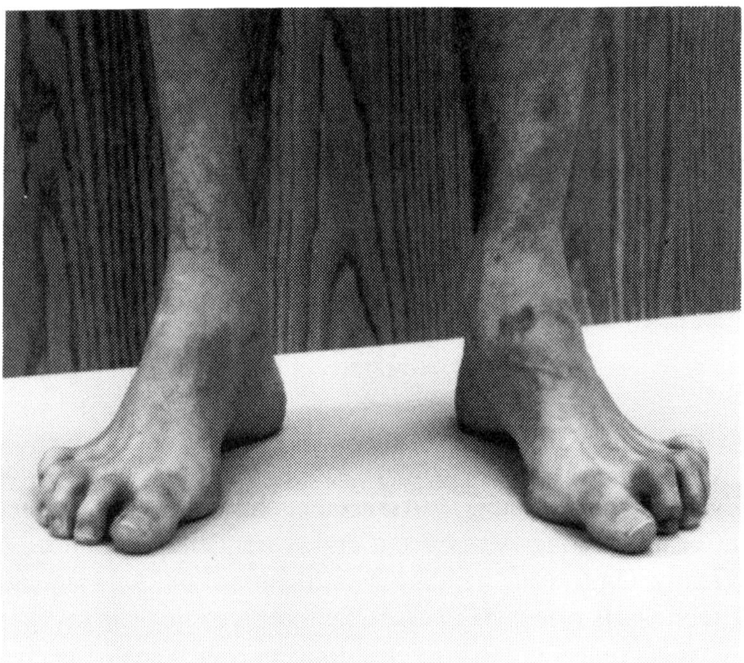

Fig. 1 Feet showing high arch and hammer toes. Left foot has been rebalanced by tendon transfer surgery.

Hands and Fingers

Wasting of the hand muscles generally leads to progressive clumsiness of the fingers. Before the muscle atrophy is seen in the hypothenar eminence (the side of the palm opposite the thumb), and at the base of the fingers, CMT patients generally adapt their activities. For instance, they have trouble with the handling of small objects such as coins and pills, but they make adaptations for it. They also adapt their movements, dressing, and shoe lace tying, and are seen to use clothing that snaps or has Velcro fastenings instead of buttons and shoe laces. Also, grasping can become difficult. They try not to carry heavy objects, or they compensate by using the forearm for carrying short distances. Because the long finger flexors are generally functioning well, the intrinsic weakness in the hand muscles can result in muscle imbalance and the development of flexion contractures of the fingers. Thumb opposition can also be compromised. Sensory changes may give a tingling or burning sensation to the fingers, but since these changes come on very gradually and subtly, the patients usually adapt readily. Figure 2 (a) and (b) show the hand of a Charcot-Marie-Tooth patient, 16 years of age with muscle atrophy in the palm and flexion contracture of the fingers. This can be improved by stretching.

Spine

The spine is affected in patients with CMT neuropathies, especially when the weakness is first seen in childhood. The development of mild scoliosis can occur and is frequently unnoticed by the family. On forward bending, prominence of one side indicates that scoliosis is present (Figure 3). School screening can reveal an atypical curve leading to a referral to a children's scoliosis clinic or to a pediatric orthopedist. Scoliosis, kyphosis, and

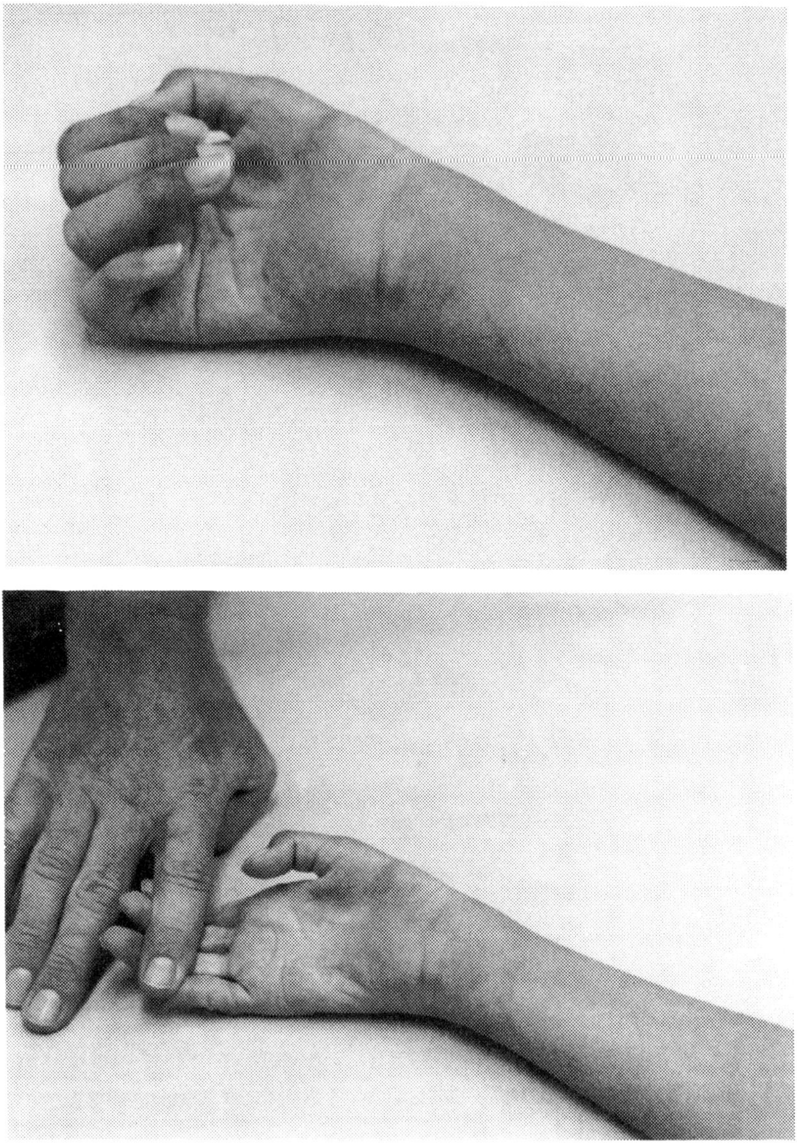

Fig.2(A) Attitude of the hand showing muscle wasting and flexion contractures of the fingers. (B) Contractures can be improved by stretching.

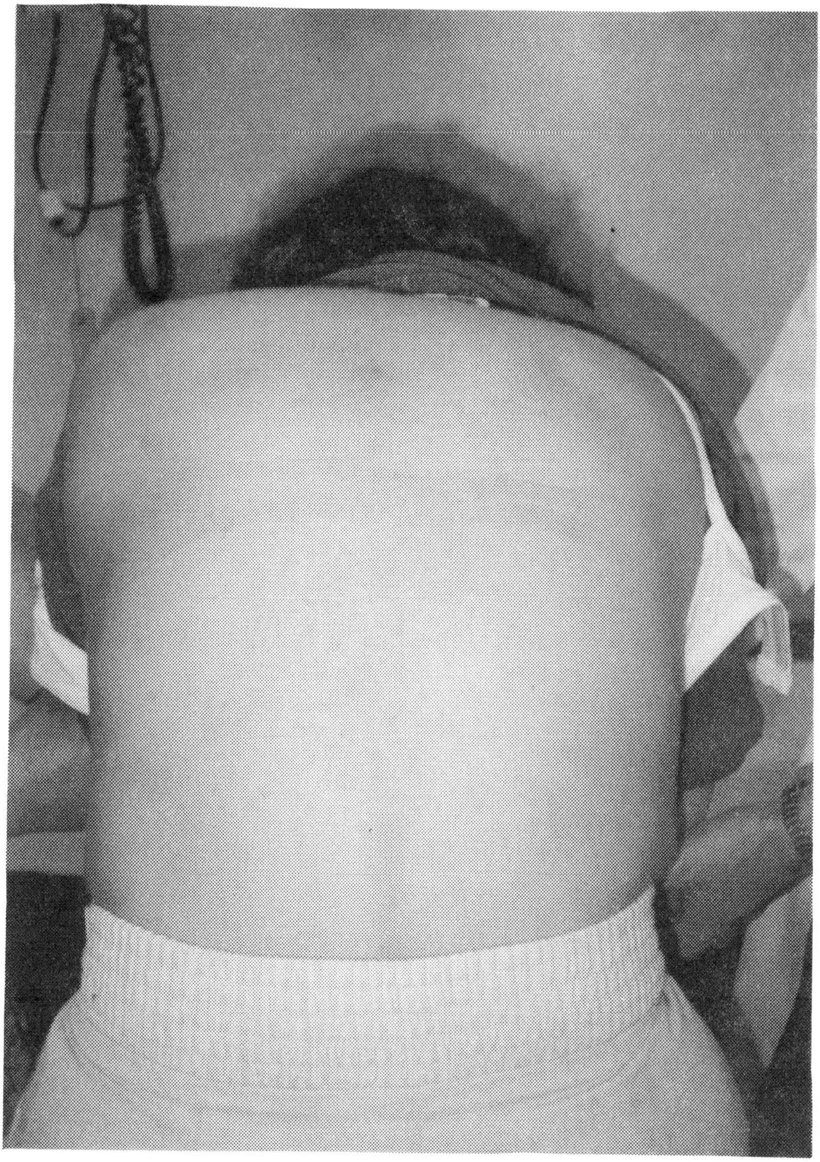

Fig.3 Mild scoliosis demonstrated by forward bending

kyphoscoliosis can also occur before hand and feet symptoms are noticed by the patient and family (2).

Hip Dysplasia

Although uncommon, patients who have difficulty walking, and have hip weakness and pain, should be examined for hip dysplasia. It is most commonly seen in patients when the disease manifests early and there are severe foot and ankle deformities. Hip dysplasia could lead to progressive hip subluxation and the development of arthritis. This condition needs to be recognized and is most usually confirmed by x-ray examination. Appropriate treatment measures can be instituted to prevent pain and further deterioration (3).

Treatment

Foot and ankle deformities represent the most common problem for CMT patients, leading them to seek orthopedic or orthotic care. Thus, this represents an area where major treatment development has been focused.

Ankle and Foot Sprains

Ankle sprains tend to occur when a CMT patient with ankle weakness walks on uneven ground and experiences sudden eversion or inversion movements. Generally, the ligaments of the ankle together with the joint capsule and musculature do a good job of supporting the ankle. However, after frequent such insults, the ankle ligaments become weakened and allow the joint to swell. Ligament laxity can lead to instability. Therefore, when an ankle sprain occurs, treatment should be made as soon as possible. First aid treatment should include ice packs around the ankle, not bearing weight, wrapping the foot and ankle with a supportive elastic bandage, and using crutches. After the acute phase is over, if the sprain is severe, a short-leg walking cast may be indicated. Sprains need to be taken seriously, since frequent recurrence of sprains will lead to ligament laxity and further instability. High top shoes or boots may serve as a reasonable preventive measure.

Ankle and Foot Muscle Imbalance

Frequently, the foot turns because peroneal muscles weaken before other muscles. Ankle and foot become imbalanced because the anterior and posterior tibials remain strong. The person starts walking on the outside of the heel and foot. Initially, the supple deformity can be supported by an orthosis such as a Berkeley Shell (UCB) or a lightweight polypropylene ankle foot orthosis (AFO). With the progression of the weakness, further imbalance occurs and the brace no longer is effective. Walking on the outside of the foot produces ; thus, a rebalancing orthopedic procedure may be indicated. The posterior tibial tendon, the tendon that is causing the abnormal pull, may need to be rerouted anteriorly through the interosseus membrane and reattached to the dorsum of the foot (4,5). Failure to do so and allowing the foot to remain unbalanced can lead to severe, permanent deformities. (Figure 4)

Fixed foot and ankle deformity resulting in contractures will occur when there is long-standing muscle imbalance. The plantar ligament and fascia at the bottom of the foot contract. Further muscle pull on the dorsum of the foot leads to the creation of a high arch (pes cavus). Further weight bearing on abnormal areas of the foot leads to callus formation and pain.

When permanent foot deformities are present, treatment can no longer be limited to the soft tissues. The underlying bone needs to be corrected to reposition the foot in a plantigrade fashion. Osteotomy of the calcaneus to reposition the heel, if this is the main cause of the deformity, is a frequently used orthopedic procedure.

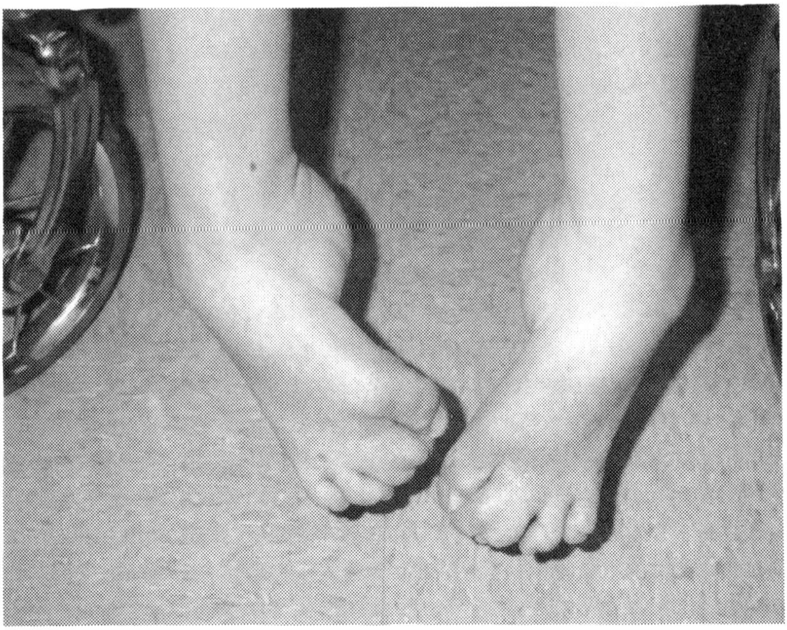

Fig.4 Severe residual fixed foot and ankle deformities with strong unopposed posterior tibial musculature.

When the deformity involves several hindfoot bones, then a triple arthrodesis becomes the surgical procedure of choice (6).

Forefoot

In the high arch, imbalance in the toe flexor tendons may cause a further abnormal pull, leading to the formation of hammer toes. The hammer toes may be tolerable but their rubbing on the shoes may cause abnormal on the top and end of the toes. Appropriate local measures include paring, splinting, padding, and shoe relief. However, if these are persistent, then toe surgery in the form of inter-phalangeal fusion, rebalancing of the tendons, and cutting the tendon that is causing the abnormal pull may all be indicated.

Hand Procedures

Hand muscle wasting and weakness usually occur later in life. Fixed flexion contractures can be treated and prevented with early appropriate stretching and splinting. However, when flexion contractures occur, releases can be made surgically, but usually the contractures recur. If thumb opposition has been lost, occasionally an opponensplasty may be indicated. This operation helps pull over the thumb by rerouting the tendon of the fourth finger to the thumb.

Spine

The spine needs to be carefully watched and severe scoliosis or kyphoscoliosis prevented. Scoliosis generally produces a rib hump when a person bends, and if this deformity is noticed, treatment needs to be started. Back exercises may be indicated at an early phase, but if necessary, bracing by the use of a containment type of body jacket may help. When spinal curvatures become severe, spinal fusion is indicated.

Hip

Hip dysplasia occurs in about 10% of CMT patients. When hip pain occurs in young adults, radiographs of the hip need to be taken. Appropriate treatment measures include the use of anti-inflammatory medication. Severe hip dysplasia may require operative treatment.

Summary

The primary care physician is an integral member of the treatment team for the CMT patient. Early recognition of orthopedic problems allows for treatment before fixed deformities occur and helps prevent pain and disability.

References

1 Sabir M., Lyttle D. Pathogenesis of pes cavus in Charcot-Marie-Tooth Disease. *Clin. Ortho. Rel. Res.*: 175:173-178, 1983.

2 Hensinger R.N.,MacEwen G.D. Spinal deformity associated with heritable neurological conditions:Spinal muscular atrophy, Friedrich's Ataxia, Familia Dysautonomia and Charcot-Marie-Tooth Disease *J.Bone Joint Surg.*, 58A;13-24, 1976.

3 Pailthorpe C.A., Benson M.K.D'A. Hip Dysplasia in hereditary motor and sensory neuropathies. *J.Bone Joint Surg.* ; 74B:538-540, 1992.

4 Hsu J.D., Hoffer M.M. Posterior tibial tendon transfer anteriorly through the interosseous membrane. *Clin.Ortho. Rel. Res.*; 131:202-204, 1978.

5 Hsu J.D. Orthopaedic Care for Children and Adolescents with Charcot-Marie-Tooth Disease. In: Lovelace R.E., Shapiro H.K. Charcot-Marie-Tooth Disorders. Pathophysiology, Molecular Genetics, and Therapy. New York, Wiley-Liss, 1990.

6 Mann D.C., Hsu J.D. Triple Arthrodesis in the treatment of fixed cavovarus deformity in adolescent patients with Charcot-Marie-Tooth Disease. *Foot and Ankle* ; 13: 1-6, 1992.

FOOT AND LEG MANIFESTATIONS OF CHARCOT-MARIE-TOOTH DISORDERS

Gerald A. Weber, D.P.M.

Co-Chief Podiatric Medicine and Surgery
Cabrini Medical Center
Affiliated with the New York Medical College, New York, NY
Attending staff Department of Neurology, Neurological Institute,
Columbia Presbyterian Medical Center, New York, NY

Key words: *CMT, cavus foot, peripheral neuropathy, pathomechanics*

Foot deformities (with or without intercurrent symptomatology) are quite often the initiating factor in the diagnostic process for Charcot-Marie-Tooth (CMT) disorder. Regardless of the type of CMT, the evolution of a cavus (high arch) foot deformity is the rule rather than the exception. While not pathognomonic of CMT, pes cavus is, however, typically seen in conjunction with an underlying neurologic deficit, whether clinically overt or covert. The cavus foot deformity has been often described as a clinical hallmark feature of the disease, but is not the only compensatory neurogenic change. As many as 10 - 15% of patients with CMT actually manifest signs of pes planus (flat foot) deformity. Additional lower extremity abnormalities found in association with CMT disease include: further structural deformities; biomechanical deficits; chronic sprains; tendon contractures and inflammatory conditions of its sheath; dermatologic presentations (including but not limited to toenail deformities and ulcerations); secondary nerve entrapments; and the predisposition for traumatic conditions leading to potential fractures, dislocations, and sprains.

This chapter is intended to familiarize the physician with the more salient lower extremity manifestations of Charcot-Marie-Tooth disease, their respective forms of pathogenesis, indications for referral and consultation, and management.

Lower Extremity Disorders Found in Association with, or as a Result of, Charcot-Marie-Tooth Disorders

Orthopedic Presentations

- **Cavus Foot Deformity**

The cavus (high arch) foot type (Figure 1) is among the most common and early associated findings in patients with CMT disease. This foot type typically becomes conspicuous within the first decade of life in patients with CMT Type 1, and as early as the second and third decades of life in other types of the disease. Pes cavus in CMT is usually bilateral.

There are some variations in the cavus foot deformity seen with CMT, with the underlying pathogenesis and potential sequelae of these variant presentations holding particular significance. For example, the cavus foot may be either a global cavus,with the apex or breech of the structural defect occurring uniformly across the midfoot region from medial to lateral, (Figure 2); a local deformity,with the apex of the deviation being to the first (ray) metatarsal and/or corresponding medial cuneiform bone, (Figure 3); or a combination of the two deformities entailing global distribution with disproportionate greater plantarflexion involvement of the first metatarsal. A pure global deformity, seen later in the course of the disease, appears to be the more prevalent.

Additional structural variations of the cavus foot deformity include a varus (inverted) deformity of the heel or the forefoot (often

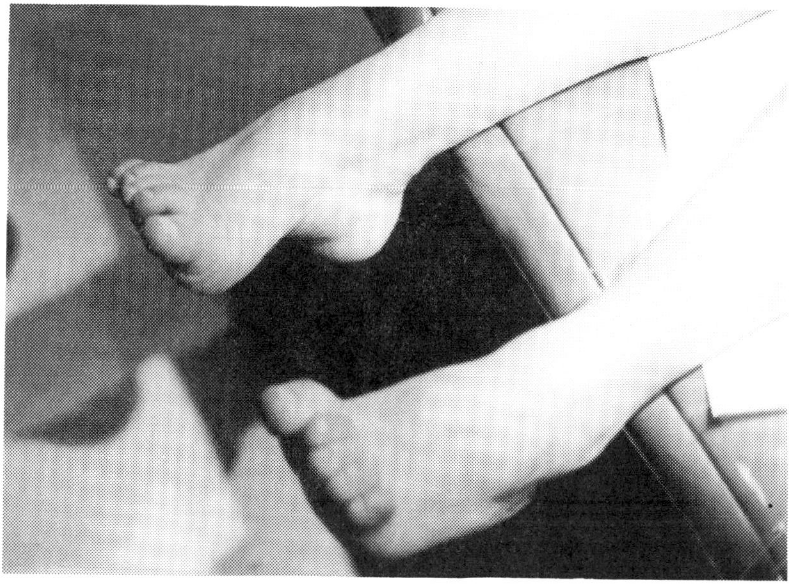

Fig. 1. The cavus or high arch foot type which is characteristic in this disorder.

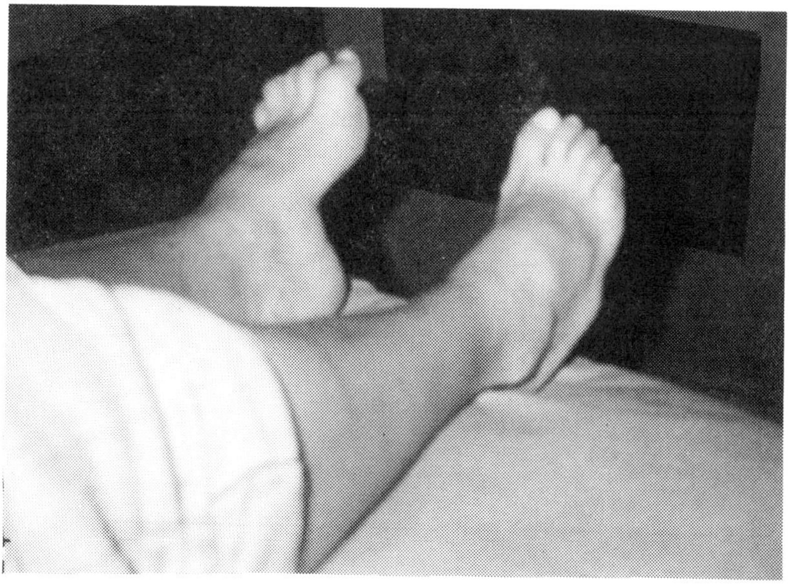

Fig. 2. Global cavus foot type

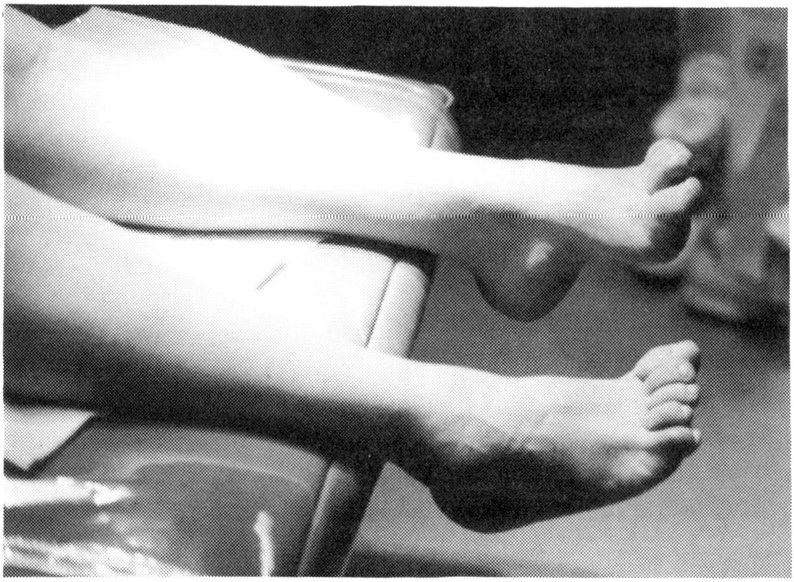

Fig. 3. Anterior local cavus foot type

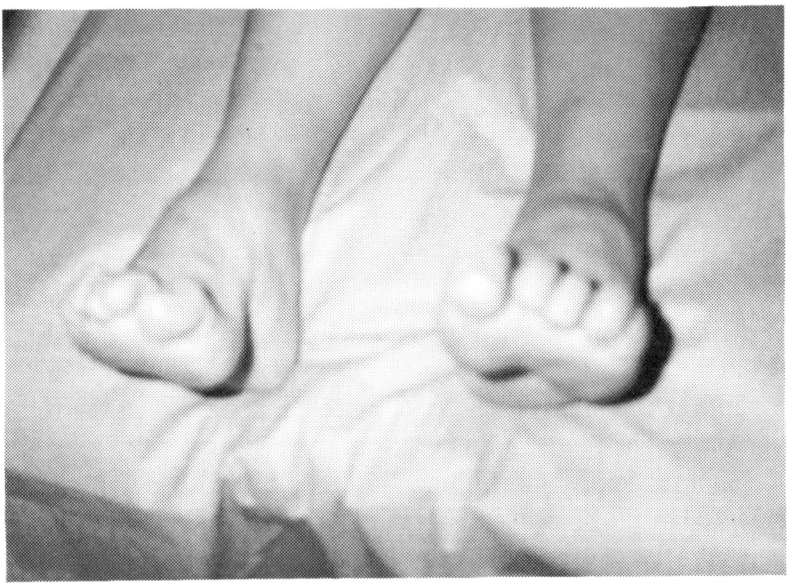

Fig. 4. Atrophied or anteriorly displaced metatarsal fat pad

appearing inverted and abducted). This will be superimposed upon a global or local cavus foot deformity.

The most consistent pathogenic factor in all structural deformities is muscle imbalance induced by the underlying neuropathy. However, other variables such as the patient's congenital structural development, interposed trauma, and the impact of other disorders upon the skeletal system, need to be recognized.

Symptoms associated with the cavus foot deformity include pain under the ball of the foot due to excessive callus formation and bursitis, as a result of an atrophied and displaced plantar metatarsal fat pad (Figure 4). There is also pain in the arch or heel due to strained or inflamed plantar fascia (plantar fascitis), with or without intercurrent bursitis. Pain along the dorsal or dorsa-lateral aspect of the foot due to a tenosynovitis (with or without accompanying bursitis) of the extensor tendons of the foot, can also occur. The last is particularly seen in the peroneus brevis tendon along the dorso-lateral aspect of the foot and ankle. This occurs especially with intercurrent adducto-varus deformity of the foot and may be related to ankle instability.

Clinical findings associated with the cavus foot deformity include bilateral high arched feet with the forefoot plantarflexed with respect to the rearfoot, and the first metatarsal being conspicuously plantarflexed. Additional findings include a varus (inverted) heel noted either during stance or non-weightbearing, with an inability to evert the heel by the examiner. (Figure 5) Likewise, the forefoot may appear abducted and inverted in relationship to the rearfoot (Figure 6). The digits in this last foot type will typically present with hammer deformities (Figure 7). The sole of the foot will often be marked by the presence of a taut, contracted band of underlying connective tissue,especially in the later stages of the disease, being most prominent medially about the arch region. The plantar

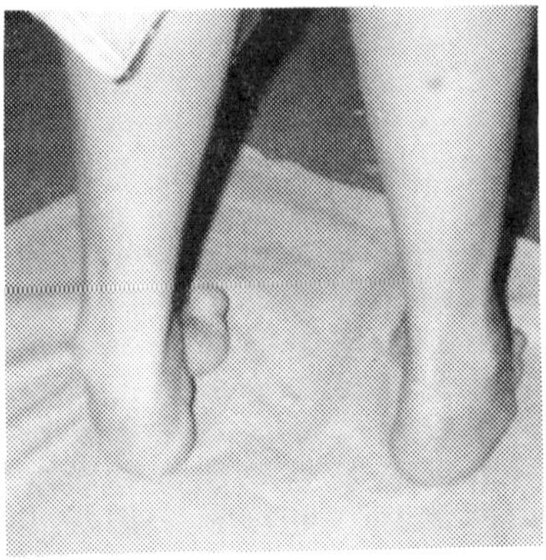

Fig. 5. Varus heel

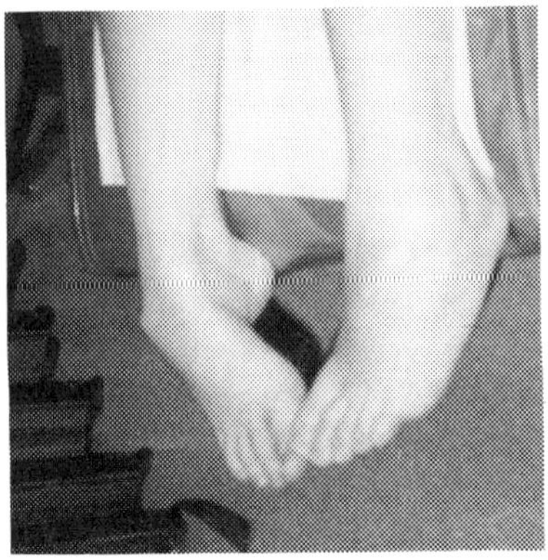

Fig. 6. Abducted inverted forefoot

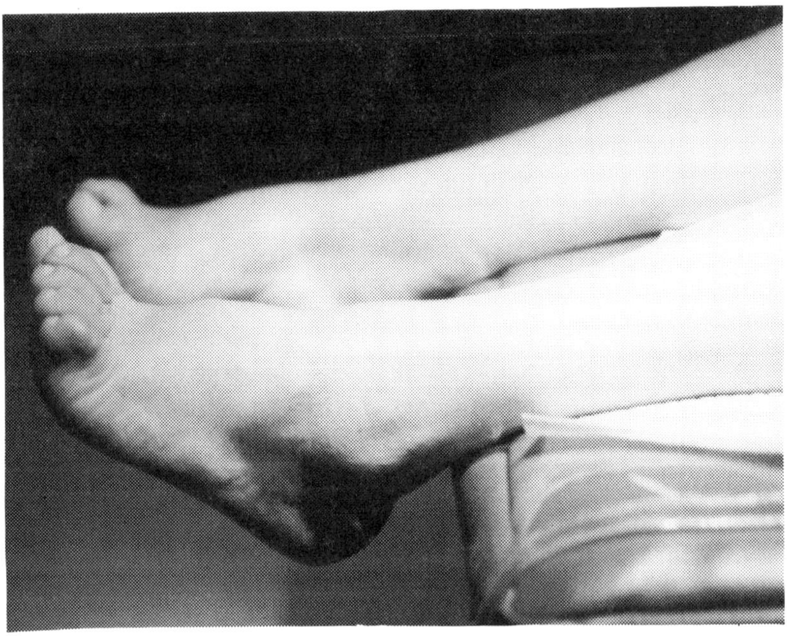

Fig. 7. Hammer digit deformities

metatarsal fat pad is apt to be atrophied and anteriorly displaced after the third decade of life in all forms of the disease. Calluses may appear along the lateral border of the heel, diffusely under the ball of the foot, as well as at the base of the fifth metatarsal and on the dorsum of the digits. The intrinsic musculature of the foot characteristically atrophies early in the course of the disease. All of the extrinsic tendons of the foot can become contracted. These contractures are directly related to the weakness, and are greatest with the widest difference of weakness between agonist and antagonist muscles (eg., severe peroneus brevis weakness with well preserved tibialis posterior muscle function). Additional clinical findings include limited ankle and subtalar joint range of motion.

Treatment of the cavus foot deformity may be divided into either a palliative, functional control, or structural surgical intervention.

Palliative measures are essentially directed at immediate relief of acute discomfort and/or inflammation. This often entails debridement of regions of excessive callus formation with dispersion padding.Other palliative modes of care may include physical therapy (eg., connective tissue massage) although certain procedures (eg., heat) may be contraindicated with severe sensory loss. Injection of local anesthetics and semi-soluble steroids may help during acute episodes, such as bursitis. Oral nonsteroidal anti-inflammatory medications are much less effective;if needed for long periods, an inflammatory cavus disorder should be suspected. Palliative measures usually give only temporary relief and other treatments will usually be needed eventually.

Various forms of toe splints, orthotics, or braces are usually highly effective in the amelioration of secondary structural deformities of the foot, while simultaneously enhancing the function of the patient. Toe splints (Figure 8) may slow the development of the secondary hammer toe deformities often seen in association

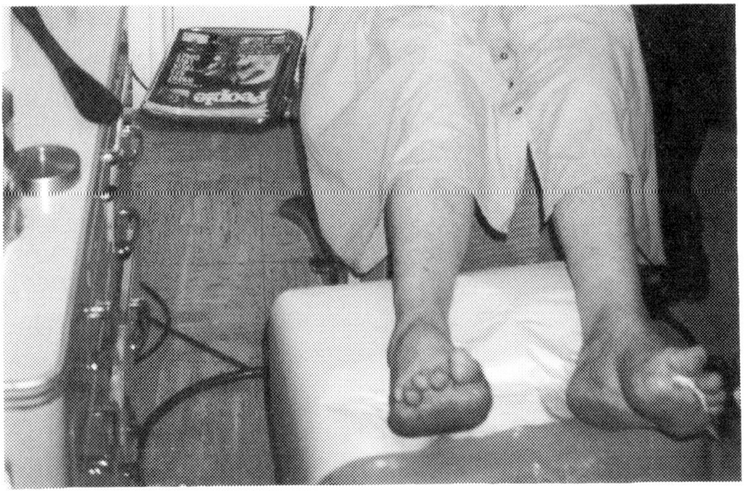

Fig. 8. Toe Splints

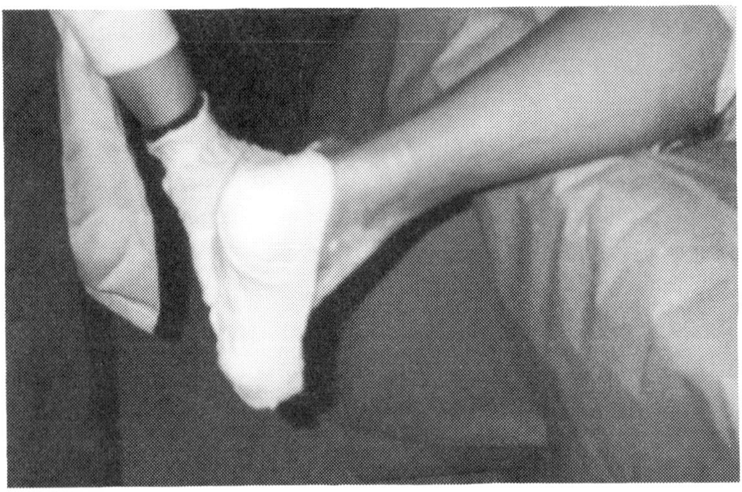

Fig. 9. Custom accommodative orthoses

with cavus foot deformities, and thus minimize painful callus conditions and bursitis. Custom orthoses (Figure 9) for the foot are highly effective in symptomatic relief of heel and forefoot disorders associated with the cavus foot deformity and also retard progression of these structural deformities. As more proximal muscles become weak, various braces (eg., PlO, molded ankle foot orthosis) will become necessary to maintain ambulation and reduce the risk of falling. Appropriate bracing will significantly limit the progression of tendon contractures and skeletal deformities, in addition to enhancing function. Once pronounced skeletal deformities have occurred, surgery may be needed for symptomatic relief, to improve function and to obtain proper fitting of the patient's foot in a brace (Figure 10). Commonly performed surgical procedures for cavus foot deformity include: osteotomies of the first metatarsal, midfoot and calcaneus; arthroplasties or arthrodesis of the digits; tendon lengthening; exostectomies; and on rare occasions, fusion of the larger joints of the foot.

Sequelae of inadequately treated cavus foot deformity in CMT disease include ankle sprains, fractures of the foot and ankle (or even other bones of the body due to instability leading to falls, dislocations, contractures, tenosynovitis, traumatic arthritis, premature degenerative joint disease, pathologic fractures, focal nerve entrapments, blisters and ulcerations with or without sinus tracts.) This last condition could lead to osteomyelitis.

The referral of a CMT patient with cavus foot deformity to a podiatrist, well experienced in the management of neuromuscular conditions afflicting the foot, could be both therapeutic and preventive. Therapy of intercurrent dermatologic, neurologic, vascular and orthopedic complications should be coordinated.

- **Pes Planus Deformity**

A much smaller number of patients with CMT may actually present with pes planus (flatfoot). Patients with pes planus may appear to have a high arch in a non-weightbearing state, only to demonstrate little or no medial arch upon full weightbearing (Figure 11). CMT patients with this foot type have more denervation of peroneus brevis than tibialis posterior. However, additional factors such as congenital predisposition to this foot type and trauma may also play a role.

Symptoms associated with the pes planus foot deformity commonly include burning or cramping along the sole of the foot,usually in the arch region but also involving the heel, cramping of the digits and calves, painful calluses under the ball of the foot, pain emanating from the point of insertion of the tibialis posterior (plantar-medial midfoot region) and less often the insertion of the peroneus brevis (base of the fifth metatarsal) often radiating proximally along the tendon sheath(s), and medial ankle instability.

Clinical findings associated with the pes planus foot deformity include the following: a minimal or absent medial arch upon full weight bearing on the foot, relative degrees of a hallux valgus (bunion) deformity, hammer toe deformities, exostosis (bone proliferation) of the medial aspect of the midfoot, callus along the ball of the foot (either discrete or diffusely), tendon contractures (the peroneus brevis and achilles often being the most conspicuous), pain on direct palpation of the plantar surface of the calcaneus (less often posteriorly) due to plantar fascitis or achilles tenosynovitis with or without bursitis and spur formation, and often, limited range of motion of the ankle, subtalar and first metatarsal-phalangeal joints.

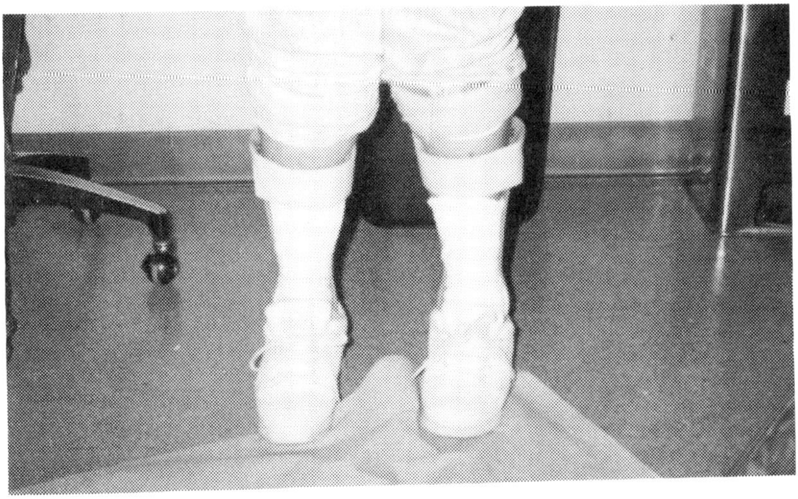

Fig. 10. Brace

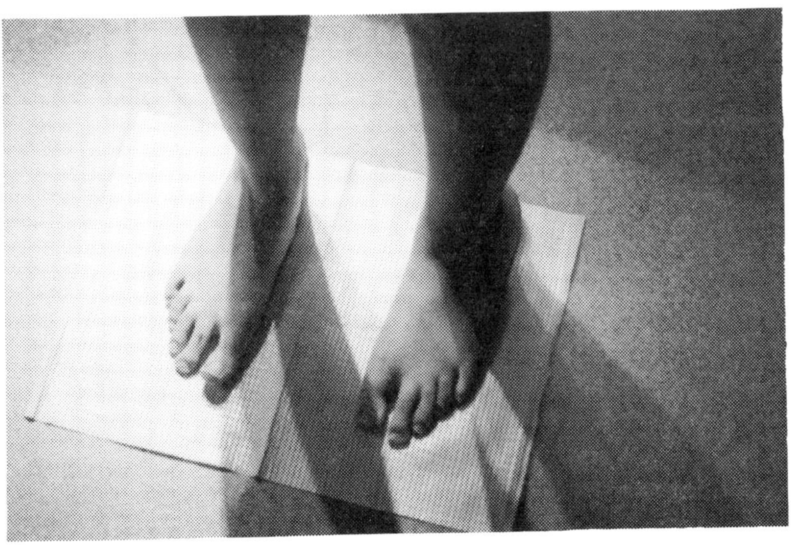

Fig. 11. Pes planus or flat foot type

Treatment of pes planus deformity in CMT may again be divided into either palliative, functional control or surgical measures, as described for cavus foot deformities. Palliative care may involve debridement of the callus with dispersion padding, debridement of toenails, physical therapy and anti-inflammatory agents. Once again the role of palliative care is invariably short-lived, and long-term therapy should focus on retarding, if not correcting, the underlying deformities.

Toe splints, foot orthoses and ankle-foot orthoses can control progression of the deformities and alleviate symptoms. Such aids need to be individualized for the pes planus foot deformity and are more useful when controlling undesirable or excessive motion (Figure 12). Molded ankle-foot orthoses will often be more helpful in preventing concurrent medial and lateral ankle joint instability.

Surgery may be considered when discomfort is not relieved with palliative and orthotic measures, or the risk of secondary sequelae is too great and the deformity is unresponsive to conservative measures alone. Furthermore, the development of certain deformities (eg., heel cord contracture, bone deformities) may preclude proper fitting within a brace without appropriate surgery.

Sequelae found in association with an untreated or inappropriately treated CMT patient with pes planus foot deformity include ankle sprains, traumatic fractures, pathologic (stress) fractures, dislocations, contractures, tenosynovitis, traumatic and/or premature osteoarthritis, focal nerve entrapment (particularly within the tarsal tunnel region) syndromes, blisters, dystrophic skin and nail charges, and ulcerations with or without contiguous osteomyelitis.

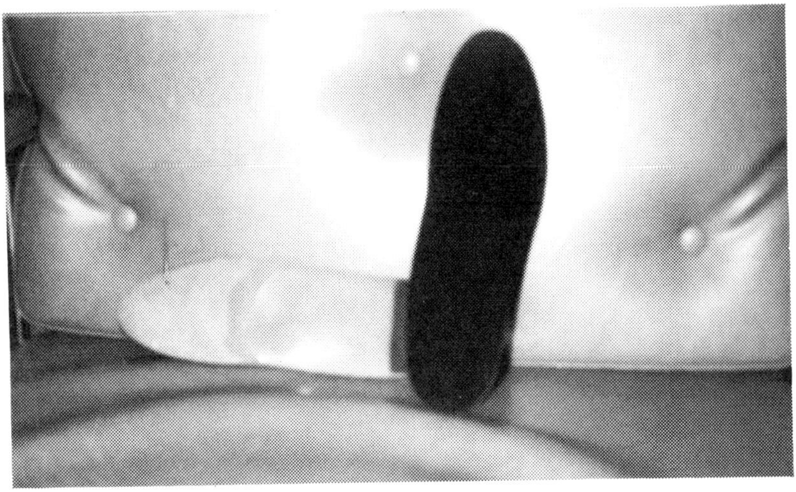

Fig. 12. Orthoses

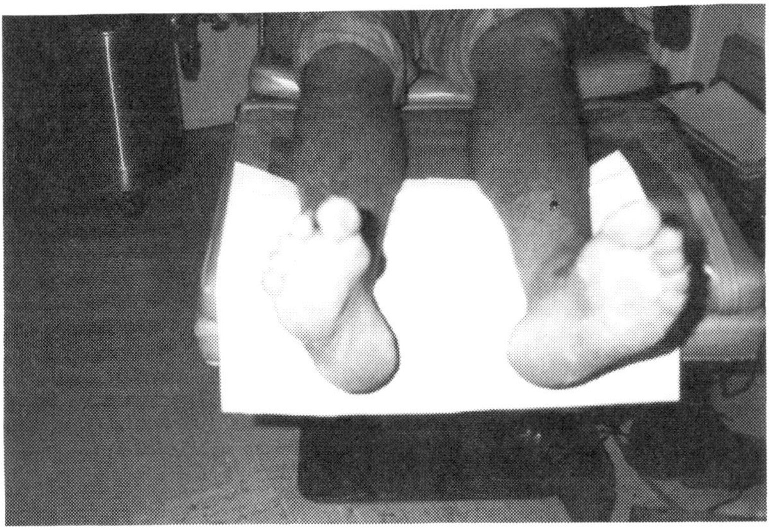

Fig. 13. Xerosis

- **Secondary Orthopedic Deformities Found To Evolve in Foot Types Associated With CMT Disease**

As previously mentioned, exostoses (bone spurs) can develop. These form over the dorsal aspect of the first metatarsal-cuneiform joint and the base of the fifth metatarsal in patients with a cavus foot type and over dorsal or medial aspect of the first metatarsal head, as well as along the plantar medial aspect of the navicular in the pes planus foot deformity.They also occur in the region of the calcaneus (most plantar and posterior aspects) in either foot type. Acute episodes of inflammation associated with such bony prominence usually respond quite well to a series of analgesic/steroid injections, in conjunction with immobilization. Physical therapy and oral non-steroidal agents appear to be less effective. Follow-up treatment with orthoses is often very successful in preventing recurrence. In situations in which patients remain resistant to such measures or are liable to secondary ulceration or chronic synovitis, surgical intervention may be necessary.

Degenerative joint disease frequently occurs when pedal joints have been malaligned for a prolonged period of time. Though all joints are at risk, the most functional articulations (ankle, subtalar, midtarsal and first metatarsal-phalangeal) are affected most often. Early implementation of proper physical therapy (eg., stretching, tone enhancement) and orthotic/bracing devices may delay premature osteoarthritis. Once again, should all conservative measures fail, or the likelihood for further compensator sequelae increase, surgery may be necessary.

Stress fractures may develop and bone disease becomes particularly noteworthy where the sensory deficit is pronounced. Fractures may also occur if the structural malalignment of the bones is due to severe muscle imbalance. The treatment entails non-weightbearing cast immobilization. However, due to pre-existing demineralization and pronounced distal muscle atrophy, prolonged immobilization may result in greater risk of fractures, fibrosis and contractures. In such instances, simultaneous incorporation of bone and muscle stimulators (extrinsically) into the cast, until adequate healing occurs, permits a return to gradual weightbearing.

II. Soft Tissue Conditions of the Foot and Leg Associated with CMT Disorders

- **Tenosynovitis**

Patients with CMT will often have at least one episode of inflammation of the tendon sheath of various extrinsic muscles of the foot regardless of their predominant foot type. Such an occurrence is due to a significant muscle imbalance between the affected muscle and its stronger antagonist which is induced by the underlying neurogenic process. Patients may respond to injection therapy in conjunction with immobilization, with or without muscle relaxants and oral non-steroidal agents, followed by physical therapy and an appropriate orthosis. However, if the affected tendon inserts into a bony prominence it usually becomes progressively hypertrophied over time. Surgical intervention may then be required to eliminate what otherwise results in a painful recalcitrant and disabling condition entailing tenosynovitis, bursitis, and a periostitis.

- **Bursitis**

Anatomical bursae are numerous and normally reside between bones, bones and tendons as well as between tendons, serving to buffer friction and pressure. However, due to the various structural and functional disturbances of the foot in patients with CMT, excessive pressure and friction is apt to result, causing bursitis.

Regardless of the sites where such a condition may arise, the patient usually responds most quickly to injection therapy. Immobilization, through casting may also be required. Again, depending on the severity and location of the bursitis, physical therapy (eg., ultrasound) may be equally effective. Follow-up therapy with an appropriate orthotic will usually safeguard against recurrence. A podiatrist well experienced in neuromuscular disorders of the foot can select and time the phases of treatment for bursitis, and is conversant with the many anatomical bursae of the foot. Adventitious (not normally occurring in that region) bursae may form as well, usually superficially in response to dermal friction, and result in secondary bursitis.

- **The Polyneuropathy of CMT**

Direct effects on the foot of the neuropathy (eg., weakness, instability, numbness and paresthesia) are commonly encountered. Physical therapy, in conjunction with appropriate orthoses, are effective in offsetting both the perception and sequelae of weakness and instability in the patient with CMT. Paresthesia, (eg. "pins and needles" or burning), though not as common nor as overt as motor symptoms, may often respond to orthotic therapy alone, or in conjunction with physical therapy.Capsaicin cream may help burning pain. If the sensory symptoms are particularly severe, walking barefoot or using thermal medicinal agents should be avoided.

- **Focal Nerve Entrapment Syndromes**

Peripheral nerves are at risk of entrapment in CMT. Entrapment may arise due to direct trauma (eg., traction), indirect trauma (eg., edema, hematoma, fibrosis), foot deformities (eg., excessive pronation in a pes planus foot deformity causing compression of the nerves within the tarsal tunnel region), or as a result of a space-occupying lesion (eg., exostosis, ganglion cyst induced by a chronic synovitis condition). Patients with CMT disease are particularly susceptible to entrapment syndromes, as the nerves are already compromised. Any associated weakness and instability from the general condition creates a greater risk of trauma and pathomechanical dysfunction. Aside from potential involvement of the common peroneal nerve at the level of the fibular neck, other nerves at risk include the sural, intermediate dorsal cutaneous (particularly following an inversion sprain), saphenous, posterior tibial and its medial and lateral plantar divisions (associated with various etiologies of tarsal tunnel syndrome), and even the common digital nerves. Clinical signs and symptoms will usually reveal disproportionate findings of sensory or motor disturbance within the distribution of the affected nerve. Electrodiagnostic studies may confirm disproportionate involvement of the afflicted nerve. Treatment is dependent upon the nerve affected, location of the entrapment, etiology, duration of the condition and the underlying status of the patient. Various forms of therapy (eg., physical therapy, injection, immobilization, surgical decompression) may significantly relieve symptoms. However, as previously discussed, the additional neural compromise is usually irreversible.

- **Edema**

Edema,when it occurs, becomes a chronic and indolent process due to the lack of functional extrinsic pedal musculature, which generally assists peripheral hemodynamics. The skin in the affected area will need supportive hydrating emollient creams due to compromised turgor. The use of custom prescribed support stockings or daily compression boot therapy, in absence of contraindicated systemic disorders (eg., congestive heart failure), will usually be the most effective treatment.

III. Dermatologic Conditions Associated With CMT Disease

- **Xerosis (dry skin)**

Xerosis (Figure 13) is usually seen only in those patients with a moderate-severe sensory impairment. The goal of therapy is to prevent skin breakdown (eg. fissures, ulcerations) and resultant infections. A moisturizing emollient is the treatment of choice.

- **Dystrophic Toenails**

As sensory denervation becomes pronounced, the structures it supplies become affected. The toenails (particularly the hallux) may, therefore, become dystrophic (Figure 14), manifested as thickening and incurvation of all affected toenails. This results in pain and secondary infection (paronychia).CMT patients should receive regular palliative therapy and avoid cutting their own toenails. If infections persist and become chronic, surgical nail avulsion with excision of the matrix (nail root) is recommended. Extreme caution against the use of chemical agents to destroy the nail matrix, particularly in patients with pronounced sensory loss or immunologic compromise, cannot be overly emphasized.

- **Blisters**

Pedal friction may cause blisters in CMT patients, particularly those with sensory loss. The blister should never be deroofed. Using sterile and aseptic technique, it should be drained and the lesion should then be dressed with an appropriate topical agent and a dry sterile dressing. The blister should heal within 2-3 weeks and subsequent attention should then be directed toward the provision of appropriate shoewear, orthotics with coverings to prohibit friction, and avoiding a particular activity by the patient which may accentuate the risk for recurrence.

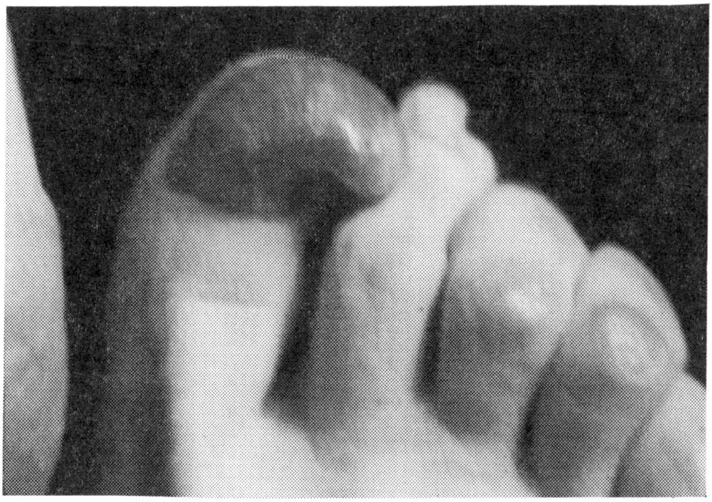

Fig. 14. Dystrophic nails

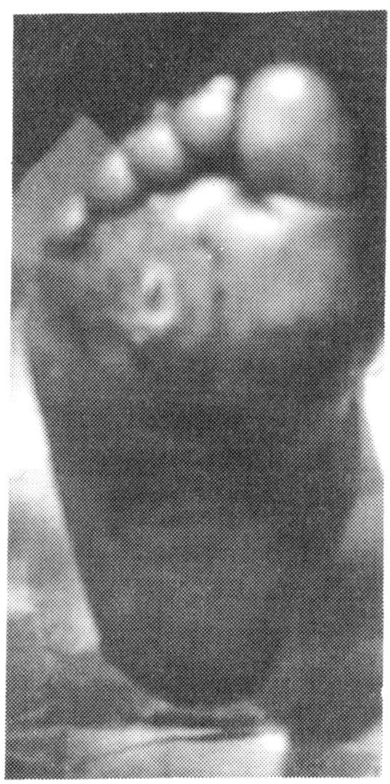

Fig. 15. Neurotrophic ulcer

- **Neurotrophic Ulcerations**

While rare in patients with CMT, neurotrophic ulceration (Figure 15) may occur. Usually situated under a bony prominence (eg., first metatarsal head), these ulcers typically respond well to debridement and a variety of wound stimulating agents, in conjunction with sterile dispersion padding of the ulcer site. Appropriately designed accommodative orthoses are generally highly effective in the prevention of recurrence of the lesion. On rare occasions, surgical intervention entailing exostectomy (removal of a bony prominence) may be required in order to provide long term resolution.

Summary

The foot and leg manifestations of Charcot-Marie-Tooth disorders may be subtle in nature, particularly during the earlier periods of development. The orthopedic presentations, especially the cavus (high arched) foot deformity, are the most widely recognized. However, a major intent of this section is to familiarize physicians with other orthopedic presentations of the disease and their forms of pathogenesis and sequelae. An additional focus addresses the need to detect involvement of the lower extremity (eg., dermatologic, neurologic) which will often reveal characteristic features as well as secondary signs and symptoms which are not directly the result of the neurogenic process.

In conclusion, it must be emphasized that early detection and referral to podiatric physicians experienced in the management of neuromuscular conditions afflicting the foot and leg, in concert with the allied disciplines responsible for health care of the CMT patient, may reduce the risk of serious complications.

References

Barrenfield P: The congenital cavus foot clin. *Orthop.*, 79:119, 1971

Bentzon PG: Pes cavus and the peroneal longus. *Acta Orthop. Scand.*, 4:50, 1933

Brewerton DA: "Idiopathic" pes cavus: an investigation into its etiology. *Br. Med. J.*, 2:659, 1963

Brooke MH: *Clinician's View of Neuromuscular Diseases*, p. 69, The Williams and Wilkens Co., Baltimore, 1977

Buchtal F, Behse F: Peroneal muscle atrophy and related diseases: clinical manifestations as related with biopsy findings, nerve conduction and electromyography. *Brain*, 99:41-66, 1976

Chapman MW, Ed.: *Operative Orthopedics* 2nd ed. J.B. Lippincott Co., Philadelphia, 1993

Cole WH: The treatment of clawfoot., *J.B.J.S.* 22:895, 1940

Dwyer FC: Osteotomy of the calcaneum for pes cavus. *J.B.J.S.* 41B:80, 1959

Fenton CF, McGlamry ED, Perrone M: Severe pes cavus deformity secondary to Charcot-Marie-Tooth disease. *J.A.P.M.A.*, 72, 4:171-175, 1982

Gould N: Surgery in advanced Charcot-Marie-Tooth disease. *Foot and Ankle*, 4, 5:267-273, 1984

Green D, Lepow GM, Smith TF: *Pes Cavus. Comprehensive Textbook of Foot Surgery.* ED McGlamary, Ed., Williams and Wildins, Baltimore, 1987

Jacobs JE, Carr CR: Progressive muscular atrophy of the peroneal type (Charcot-Marie-Tooth disease). *J.B.J.S.*, 32 A1:27-38, 1950

Jahss MH: Evaluation of the cavus foot for orthopedic treatment. *Clin. Ortho. Rel. Res.*, 181:52-63, 1983

Mann RA, Missirian J: Pathophysiology of Charcot-Marie-Tooth disease. *Clin. Orthol. Rel Res.*, 228-234,321, 1988

McGlamary ED, Ruch JA, Vigorito TF: Charcot-Marie-Tooth disease: a case report. *J.A.P.A.*, 65:347, 1975

McComas AJ: *Neuromuscular Function and Disorders*, p 238, Butterworth, Boston, 1977

Samilson RL, Dillon W: Cavus, cavovarus, and calcaneocavus. *Clin. Ortho. and Rel. Res.*, 177:125-131, 1983

Swanson AB, Brown HS, Coleman JD: The cavus foot: concepts of production and treatment by metatarsal osteotomy. Proceedings of the American Academy of Orthopedic Surgeons, *J.B.J.S.*, 48A: 1019, 1956

Tachdjian MO: *Pediatric Orthopedics*, WB Saunders Co., Philadelphia, 1972

CONSERVATIVE MANAGEMENT IN PATIENTS WITH CHARCOT-MARIE-TOOTH DISORDERS

Carol A. Oatis, P.T., Ph.D.*
Deborah Sundberg, M.S., P.T.
Christine Oliver, M.S., P.T.
Pamela Yerkes, M.S., P.T.

*Associate Professor, Department of Physical Therapy
Beaver College, Glenside, PA

Key words: *CMT, physical therapy, occupational therapy, weakness, strength, exercise, rehabilitation, adaptive equipment, deformities, orthoses*

Charcot-Marie-Tooth syndrome (CMT) is a group of inherited peripheral neuropathies leading to degenerative changes in peripheral motor and sensory nerves. The primary expression of this disorder is weakness of the distal muscles of the upper and lower limbs (1). Although this syndrome probably is the most common class of inherited neurologic disorder, many, if not most, of the patients with the disorder receive no medical intervention for their symptoms (2). Experience with patients and their families reveals a common scenario: the patient and family are told that "there is no treatment available until perhaps you need braces or a wheelchair." This misperception may result from the recognition of the disorder as progressive, generally not fatal, but also not curable (3). However, valid intervention is not necessarily limited to treatment that can alter the physiologic course of the disorder. Consideration should also be given to treatments that may alleviate the impairments and disabilities resulting from the expression of the disorder, namely the denervation of the limbs. The purpose of this chapter is to present to the primary care provider the conservative treatments available to the patient with CMT.

The difficulty in writing this chapter is the need to balance the scientific evidence with the clinical observations. Clinicians are justified, indeed urged, to seek scientific confirmation of clinical impressions. Yet there is an equally compelling need to provide the best available care to the patient. The clinician is frequently caught between a desire to provide care and a refusal to support quackery. This chapter presents what data there are to support the role of exercise and other conservative means in the treatment of patients with CMT. It also presents the rationale and general form of conservative management of patients with CMT. The reader will find that there is very little *direct* evidence to substantiate the efficacy of exercise in managing a patient with CMT. However, the reader will also find significant *indirect* support from studies which demonstrate strength and functional gains in patients with a variety of progressive neurologic disorders following exercise. It is this indirect evidence that encourages us to present the practical guidelines of conservative care while recognizing the need for continued research to validate or refute this approach.

The primary manifestation of CMT is progressive muscle weakness in the upper and lower extremities, although involvement of the muscles of the axioskeleton has also been reported. Sensory loss also occurs. Most patients identify these symptoms only as they recognize an inability to carry out some function such as running or walking on uneven surfaces. It is these resulting disabilities which lead a patient to seek help, and it is toward these disabilities that conservative management should be directed. Thus, the goal of conservative management is to maximize function.

Progressive loss of strength influences function in several ways. First, of course, some activities require a threshold level of strength. For example, normal running requires a certain level of plantar flexion strength. As weakness progresses, the patient may fail to meet that threshold and normal running will no longer be possible. Second, as strength diminishes, certain tasks take on an element of risk. For example, as ankle weakness increases, walking across a broken sidewalk may present the danger of falling with its secondary risks of sprains and fractures. Third, the progression of muscle weakness appears related to the length of the nerve. Sabir and Lyttle (4) reported that the weakness in the lower extremities first appears in the smallest muscles innervated by the longest axons of the sciatic nerve. Thus, the first appearance of weakness and its subsequent progression vary among muscle groups according to their muscle mass and axon length. This variability leads to muscle imbalances resulting in joint deformities. Deformities can themselves interfere with function, such as the varus deformities of the foot, common in CMT, which predispose the patient to ankle sprains. The deformities are frequently painful and cause still further loss of function. Muscle weakness and the resulting deformities place abnormal stress on otherwise normal joints, perhaps predisposing the patient to joint degeneration. Finally, in the presence of muscle weakness, the patient has to expend more energy to accomplish a given task while frequently having less energy to spend. Thus begins a downward spiral of functional ability.

In order to optimize function, conservative management should be directed toward the following goals:

1. maximizing strength,

2. insuring safety,

3. minimizing discomfort,

4. protecting joints, and

5. conserving energy.

These goals can be met through muscle strengthening, stretching and endurance training, the application of orthotic devices, and the judicious use of adaptive equipment. Physical and occupational therapists are educated specifically in these areas and are usually best suited to work with the primary care providers to establish a treatment regimen for the patient with CMT. Because the expression of the syndrome is so varied and the rate of progression unpredictable, any intervention must be based on a complete evaluation to establish each patient's individual status and needs.

The following presents the principles and general expectations for conservative treatment of the patient with Charcot-Marie-Tooth disorder.

Muscle Training

The effect of exercise on neuropathically weakened muscle remains debatable. Early studies of patients with poliomyelitis and Duchenne muscular dystrophy reported the existence of "overuse weakness" suggesting that exercise could actually lead to additional muscle and nerve damage (5-8). Some of these authors urged the complete avoidance of exercise beyond activities of daily living (7, 8). More recently, the appearance of post-polio syndrome has amplified the concern about exercising weakened muscles (9). In speaking to patients with CMT and their families, it has become clear to me that many patients believe that exercise will actually exacerbate neuronal deterioration. However, several controlled studies of patients with neuromuscular diseases have revealed no detrimental effects of strengthening exercises (10, 11). Of course any muscle, normal or weakened, can be damaged by excessive loads or repetitions. While the threshold for injury is presumably lowered in the weakened muscle, current evidence refutes the existence of negative effects of exercise unique to neurogenically weakened muscles. Because overuse injuries could have far more serious consequences in already compromised muscles, the patient with CMT must be instructed carefully to avoid fatigue and injury (12).

Of equal importance in determining the validity of exercise in the management of patients with CMT is the question of whether neurogenic weakness actually can be retarded or reversed by exercise. Theoretically, any muscle capable of contraction is capable of strengthening that contraction (13). However, some studies of patients with neuromuscular diseases have reported no change in strength following a training regimen (14). Yet other studies of similar patients report significant increases in muscle strength and endurance (11,14,15). Abramson and Rogoff (15) reported significant strength gains in thirteen of twenty-seven subjects with muscular dystrophy. All but one of the remaining fourteen subjects showed no improvement, with the one subject demonstrating a slight decrease in strength. Milner-Brown and Miller suggested that the effect of exercise is dependent on the pre-training strength of the muscle (16). These authors proposed that if a muscle is sufficiently weak and it is functioning at a maximal level during activities of daily living, further strengthening cannot be expected from additional exercise. They also noted that the greatest improvements in strength occurred in muscles with mild to moderate weakness. These authors used their findings to urge early strengthening programs for patients with progressive neuromuscular disease.

It must be noted that the studies cited above did not specifically include patients with CMT, although not all of the authors described their sample populations. Since CMT is progressive, it is impossible to predict the degree of success of an exercise program. Exercise may slow the progression of weakness in some patients; in others it might halt the progression; and in still others, exercise may result in actual strengthening. There appears to be ample evidence thus far to support the potential gains of exercise in patients with CMT.

Discussion up to this point has focused on the effects of exercise on the involved muscles. However, muscles unaffected by the disease can also benefit from exercise. Patients with CMT frequently abandon vigorous physical activity and gravitate toward a sedentary lifestyle. This decreased level of general activity can result in progressive weakness from disuse and general deconditioning. Yet compensation for the weaknesses due to CMT frequently requires greater physical exertion and greater strength in the surrounding musculature than is normally required. Thus, strengthening the normal muscles may help the patient tolerate the increased stresses resulting from the neurogenic weakness (17). The patient with CMT should be encouraged to participate in a regular program of exercise for both the involved and uninvolved muscles.

Perhaps the most frequently agreed upon issue in the muscle training literature related to neuromuscular disorders is the importance of individualized exercise programs based on the patient's specific status and the need for careful supervision. Although deleterious effects of training unique to neurologically weakened muscles are unlikely, overtraining must be avoided to prevent further damage to the muscles (9). In addition, because weakness is generally unevenly distributed throughout the limbs in CMT, the appropriate exercise intensity will vary widely among individual muscles. Therefore, each patient should undergo a complete and specific evaluation by a physical therapist. Exercises can then be prescribed to maximize each muscle's potential while minimizing further muscle imbalances. Precision and careful education are also essential to ensure that the patient is exercising the intended muscle. The patient must also be instructed in judicious progression of each exercise to avoid excessive fatigue and overuse injuries. A physical therapist should be able to prescribe appropriate exercises and educate the patient and family in ways to avoid injury (12).

Cardiovascular Training

The presence of muscle weakness may increase the energy requirements of simple activities such as walking (18). In addition, patients with CMT often demonstrate decreased cardiovascular conditioning perhaps as a result of inactivity or perhaps as an additional sequela of the syndrome. Florence and Hagberg (19) reported a difference in cardiovascular adaptation to exercise in two patients with CMT compared to patients with myopathies, with the patients with CMT demonstrating the smallest improvement in VO2 max and heart rate. Yet these authors did note that there was a positive, albeit diminished, training response in those subjects with CMT. Thus, cardiovascular or aerobic exercise can benefit the patient with CMT, improving the patient's capacity to sustain the increased energy demands of everyday activities.

Aerobic training, like strength training, must be individualized to meet the specific needs of each patient. Because CMT frequently affects the muscles of the lower extremity, walking or jogging may be unrealistic or even dangerous. Swimming or riding a stationary bicycle may be safer and more appropriate. The benefits of aerobic exercise are well documented for the general public and include decreased risk of heart disease, decreased body fat, and improved sense of well-being (20). For the patient with CMT syndrome, aerobic exercise may provide the additional benefit of improved function in daily life.

Treatment of Deformities

One result of the uneven distribution of muscle weakness about a given joint in patients with CMT is the development of joint deformities. Weakness in one muscle or muscle group in the presence of relative strength in the opposing muscle(s) allows the stronger muscle or muscle group to pull the joint, unimpeded by the opposing muscles. Typically although not always, patients with CMT have an earlier onset of weakness in the muscles of dorsiflexion than in the opposing plantar flexors. The plantar flexors are allowed to contract unopposed and become tight, forming a "plantar flexion contracture." Such deformities limit the normal movement of the joint and cause abnormal stresses to be applied to the limb and joint. In this case the patient would have difficulty keeping the heel on the ground during ambulation, thereby putting more pressure on the forefoot.

The typical hammer toe deformities associated with intrinsic muscle weakness in the foot usually result in corns where the dorsum of the toes rub in the shoe, and calluses on the plantar surface of the feet where the metatarsal heads are exposed. Such deformities are frequently quite painful, often causing the patient to decrease weight-bearing activities such as walking. Deformities also may stress adjacent joints, which may cause additional pain and contribute to further joint damage. For example, the plantar flexion contracture described above commonly applies excessive stress on the knee joint during ambulation (21).

There are no known studies which document the ability of exercise to prevent deformities. However, clinical evidence suggests that stretching exercises are useful in reducing some deformities. Like strengthening exercises, the stretching exercises must be specific and precise to lengthen the intended muscle and must be based on a thorough understanding of the status of the patient's muscles and joints.

The Role of Orthotic Devices

Orthotic devices are used most frequently to provide joint stability in the absence of adequate muscle or ligamentous stabilization. Patients with CMT syndrome commonly use ankle foot orthoses (AFOs) to stabilize the ankle during weight-bearing activities, substituting for either the dorsiflexors or plantar flexors. Such devices can improve the patient's stability and safety by reducing the risk of falls. Additionally, the orthosis may increase the efficiency of locomotion by reducing the extraneous movements necessary to compensate for ankle weakness (22).

Orthotic devices can be equally useful in the upper extremity, especially the hand. Weakness of the intrinsic muscles of the hand is a common finding in some forms of CMT and can limit the fine motor skills of the patient. Simple splints to provide thumb stability may result in significant functional improvements.

Orthotic devices have also been used successfully to relieve the stresses caused by joint deformities. Podiatrists, orthotists, and physical therapists have used foot orthoses to relieve the pressures of some foot deformities. It must be noted that the use of most orthotic devices inhibits muscle activity around the joints incorporated in the device. Such inhibition may further weaken the muscles. The benefits of increased stability, efficiency, and comfort must be weighed against the risk of increased weakness. The application of an orthosis, like other interventions, must be based on a thorough understanding of the patient's needs and condition.

The kind of device chosen will be determined by the combined input of physician, therapist, orthotist, and patient.

Adaptive Equipment

Adaptive equipment is specially designed to reduce the difficulty of everyday activities for people with disabilities. These devices run the gamut from instruments to make buttoning a shirt easier to bathtub benches. Simple devices to improve fine motor tasks may allow a secretary to remain employed while the bathtub bench may keep a patient independent in the home. Occupational therapists are usually most familiar with such devices, and several catalogs are devoted solely to such merchandise.

Experience suggests that patients and clinicians view adaptive devices as the last resort in treatment and imply a sort of failure. However, we believe that early application of this equipment can conserve a patient's strength and energy and may even prevent some functional deterioration. Again, the use of adaptive equipment should be based on the patient's individual needs identified by careful and thorough evaluation.

Intervention for the severely affected individual frequently focuses on adaptive equipment and is essential in maintaining the individual's function. As weakness progresses in the lower extremities, the use of a wheelchair can provide continued mobility. The correct choice of wheelchairs, with consideration given to size, support and adaptability, is critical to optimize a patient's mobility. Close consideration of household adaptations, such as bathtub benches, railings and ramps, is also necessary. Physical and occupational therapists are educated to evaluate the home setting and functional needs of the patient and caregiver to optimize function and facilitate care.

Guide to the Overall Plan of Conservative Care

Following a thorough evaluation, the patient and family can usually be instructed in an exercise program which can be carried out at home with occasional reassessments to modify the program as needed. The application of orthotic devices and assistive equipment can be made as the patient's condition warrants. Such intervention rarely requires prolonged or extended care by a physical or occupational therapist. Rather, the ideal pattern of care appears to consist of an extensive initial evaluation and one or two sessions to initiate an independent program of exercise. Additional visits may be necessary to evaluate equipment needs. Once a program is established, periodic reassessments may be useful to alter the program and reevaluate the patient's needs in light of changing manifestations of the progressive disorder.

Increased muscle strength, or conversely, decreased muscle weakness, appears to improve a patient's level of function. Similarly, prevention of deformities, optimizing energy utilization, and reduction of pain all are expected to improve function. However, it must be recognized that few studies have been undertaken to test these beliefs. Hoberman (6) and Vignos (14) reported functional improvements in patients with progressive muscular dystrophy following exercise. Yet almost all of the patients I have treated or met through support groups have reported that they have been told that intervention will not alter their disease. As noted earlier in this chapter, altering the disease is not the only valid goal of treatment. However, optimism and unsupported beliefs cannot justify costly health care. Consequently, further research is needed to assess the efficacy of conservative management of CMT. Pilot studies in my own clinic suggest positive responses to the interventions described in this chapter. We are now beginning controlled studies to measure the efficacy of this approach specifically in patients with CMT.

Conclusion

The most common physical manifestations of Charcot-Marie-Tooth syndrome include muscle weakness, muscle imbalance, and joint deformities. These impairments lead to a loss of function for many patients. Studies have demonstrated the ability to improve strength in patients with neuropathies. Other studies have demonstrated improved function in such patients following a prolonged exercise regimen. While few studies have demonstrated specific functional gains in patients with CMT resulting from exercise, no known studies have refuted that possibility. While further research is needed, and under way, to test the efficacy of conservative intervention in patients with CMT, present clinical knowledge supports the use of physical and occupational therapy to ameliorate the sequelae of CMT.

References

1 Daher YH, Lonstein JE, Winter RB, et al. Marie-Tooth disease. *Clin Orthop.*; 202:219-222, 1986.

2 Shapiro HK. In summation: Our current perspective and opportunities for the future. In: Lovelace RE, Shapiro HK. *Charcot-Marie-Tooth Disorders: Pathophysiology, Molecular Genetics, and Therapy*. New York. Wiley-Liss; 1990:429-437.

3 Gilroy J, Meyer JS. *Medical Neurology*. New York: Macmillan; 1979:175-235.

4 Sabir M, Lyttle D. Pathogenesis of Charcot-Marie-Tooth disease. *Clin Orthop.*;184:223-235, 1984.

5 Lovett RW. The treatment of infantile paralysis. *JAMA*. 1915;64:2118.

6 Hoberman M. Physical medicine and rehabilitation: its value and limitations in progressive muscular dystrophy. *Am J Phys Med.*; 34:109-115, 1955.

7 Bensman A. Strenuous exercise may impair muscle function inGuillain-Barre patients. *JAMA.* ; 214:468-469 1970.

8 Johnson EW, Braddom R. Overwork weakness in facioscapulo-humeral muscular dystrophy. *Arch Phys Med Rehabil*;52:333-336, 1971.

9 Agre JC, Rodriguez AA. Neuromuscular function in polio survivors. *Orthopaedics*;14:1343-1347, 1991.

10 Delateur BJ. Giaconi RM. Effect of maximal strength submaximal exercise in Duchenne muscular dystrophy. *Am J Phys Med.*; 58:26-36 ,1979.

11 McCartney N, Moroz D, Garner SH, et al. The effects of stength training in patients with selected neuromuscular disorders. *Med Sci Sports Exerc*; 20:362-368, 1988.

12 Oatis CA. Conservative management of the functional manifestations of Charcot-Marie-Tooth disease. In: Lovelace RE, Shapiro HK. *Charcot-Marie-Tooth Disorders: Pathophysiology, Molecular Genetics, and Therapy.* New York: Wiley-Liss; 1990:416-427.

13 Brooks GA, Fahey TD. *Exercise Physiology: Human Bioenergetics and its Application.* New York: Macmillan; 1985:395-425.

14 Vignos PJ, Watkins MP. The effect of exercise in muscular dystrophy. *JAMA.*;197:121-126, 1966.

15 Abramson AS, Rogoff J. Physical treatment in muscular dystrophy (abstract). Symposium on an approach to the rehabilitation of children with muscular dystrophy. *Proceedings of the 1st and 2nd Medical Conferences of MDAA.* 1953:123-125.

16 Milner-Brown HS, Miller RG. Muscle strengthening through high-resistance weight training in patients with neuromuscular disorders. *Arch Phys Med Rehabil.*; 69:14-19, 1988.

17 Delorme TL, Schwab R, Watkins AL. The response of quadriceps femoris to progressive resistance exercises in poliomyeliticpatients. *J Bone Joint Surg.*; 30A:834-847, 1948.

18 Winter DA. Energy assessments in pathologocal gait. *Physiotherapy Canada.*; 30:183-191, 1978.

19 Florence JM, Hagberg JM. Effect of training in the exercise responses of neuromuscular disease patients. *Med Sci Sports Exerc.*;16:460-465, 1984.

20 Huhn RR, Voski RV. Primary prevention programs for business and industry: role of physical therapists. *Phys Ther.*;65:1840-1844, 1985.

21 Perry J. *Gait Analysis: Normal and Pathological Function.* Thorofare, NJ: Slack, Inc.; 1992:282-283.

22 Corcoran PJ, Jebsen RH, Berngelmann GL, et al. Effects of plastic and metal braces on speed and energy cost of hemiparetic ambulation. *Arch Phys Med Rehabil.*; 51:69-77, 1970.

CHARCOT-MARIE-TOOTH DISORDERS: A SUMMARY

Lowell L. Williams, M.D.

Key words: *immune system, fatty acids, pain, diet, vitamins, pregnancy, patient management, nutrition*

This final chapter includes important aspects of the Charcot-Marie-Tooth (CMT) disorders not previously mentioned. These are the known biochemical defects of CMT, a reasonable approach to exercise in CMT, and CMT patient nutritional needs. Autoimmune abnormalities of CMT patients and their implications for CMT disease are described. Finally, general rules and responsibilities for CMT health caretakers are outlined. I write this summary as a doctor with CMT as well as one who has cared for many CMT patients. In this dual role I have experienced the many frustrations of both sides of the treatment table.

CMT Fatty Acid Metabolism and Exercise

Despite years of genetic and diagnostic research in CMT 1, the essential biochemical defects leading to its characteristic peripheral demyelination are just beginning to be identified. Biochemical abnormalities and their correction or control are the true goals of genetic studies. Recent chromosomal advances in CMT have brought science closer to discovering these mutations. Once identified, they will form the basis for prevention and ameliorative treatment of the variations of the CMT syndrome.

Early lipid studies to interpret CMT demyelination led to the discovery by Dyck and associates of low proportions of the essential fatty acid, linoleic acid, in both CMT peripheral blood and myelin (1,2). After confirming this deficiency, my coworkers and I tried to bring this fatty acid component back to normal by adding it in the form of dietary EFAMOL plus vitamin E to 20 CMT1 patients for one year. The dietary addition occurred after a 3-month blind placebo period (3,4,5). To follow possible physical changes resulting from the added fatty acids, we tested individual hand and foot strength and dexterity and measured nerve conduction velocities repeatedly during the study. Unfortunately, the 1 year's dietary supplement in these patients did not restore their blood proportions of the low fatty acid, nor were there measurable improvements in the careful, detailed physical tests of their nerve and muscle function (3,4,5).

Although no genetically altered fatty acid enzyme defect was clearly implicated in CMT (1-5), we also explored this possibility. CMT fatty acid metabolism in skin was normal when fatty acids were measured in CMT cultured skin fibroblasts (6). In contrast, the low fatty acid values in CMT blood suggested the chronic or repeated diversion of the fatty acids to other metabolic pathways. Utilization of these omega-6 fatty acids, linoleic and arachidonic acids, for the formation of immunoregulatory prostaglandin metabolites appears confirmed in further studies of CMT blood (7). This pathway is described in more detail in the section on the immune system of CMT. We concluded that fatty acid supplements could improve the common CMT complaints of dry flaky skin and/or constipation, but that they did not change neurologic function or restore myelin during one year of treatment (3,5).

It is possible, however, that adding polyunsaturated fatty acids to the CMT diet may be important to maintain the fatty acid levels necessary for the CMT patient's well-being. Low fatty acid content in CMT peripheral tissues (1-6) may be one basis for CMT muscle weakness and for the lack of the so-called "second wind" phenomena in CMT. Present in normal individuals during exercise, this late spurt of activity is thought to be an improved muscle effort achieved "beyond pain" that uses fatty acid stores in normal muscles. Since these stores appear limited in CMT muscles, it is important to warn CMT patients that they must not exercise to the extent of muscle pain. Pain experienced by the CMT patient may indicate actual destruction of muscle proteins and lead to increased and permanent muscle damage. To help the CMT family deal with inadequate muscle functions in affected children, it is often necessary to write letters to school administrators and gym teachers requesting exemptions for CMT youths from prolonged exercise and severe competitive athletic stress. It is important for the medical caretaker to include physiologic explanations to justify this inability and also to suggest substitute gym activities. Mild to moderate exercise is excellent for CMT muscles and necessary to maintain muscle tone. Swimming and bike-riding, neither of which require weight-bearing, are ideal for the CMT youngster. An absolute rule is to encourage gentle regular movement of affected limbs and to keep as active as physically possible.

Sugar Metabolism and Weight Control in CMT

Sugar metabolism may not be completely normal in all CMT patients since pyruvate (3-carbon sugar) oxidation appears defective in some (8). Many complain of fatigue and fast heart rate following a high sugar meal. In these patients a pyruvate dehydrogenase fault may be present even with a glucose tolerance test within the normal range. If these symptoms are present, a diet low in pure sugar and high in complex carbohydrates is advisable. Of course, if associated with weight loss and excessive drinking, a complete diabetic workup is in order to evaluate a possibility of associated diabetes.

A weight-loss program should be recommended for overweight CMT patients to reduce the strain on the weight-bearing joints and muscles. A regular plan of moderate meals high in meat and fiber and low in sugar appears effective. I also recommend a daily general vitamin capsule (any brand) with the option of additional fatty acid supplements.

Immune System Defects or Auto-immune Over-activation in CMT

Abnormalities of immunity toward secondary diseases appear common in CMT patients. In an early study (9) an isolated deficiency of the epithelial surface immune factor, immunoglobulin A, was found in approximately one-third of 15 CMT families studied. This defect, also often inherited, can lead to increased sinus, pulmonary, gastro-intestinal, and urinary tract infections in those individuals. In CMT patients with chronic infections of one or more of these systems, an immune system workup is indicated to identify possible abnormal immune functions. Maintenance or repeated antibiotic therapy may be necessary to control persistent epithelial surface or skin infections in some CMT patients.

Autoimmune components appear in both blood and peripheral nerve in CMT disorders (7,10,11). Several centers described an increased expression of type II histocompatibility antigens (HLA), an autoimmune reaction, in CMT peripheral nerves (10). These reactions were consistent with an increased presence of "activation" epitopes or hyperimmune surface marker expressions on CMT lymphocytes (7,10,11). Similar to other autoimmune or chronic infectious processes, the CMT hyperimmune state appears to be cyclic or periodic when examined over time (7,11). Possible destruction of peripheral nerve myelin by an autoimmune process is suggested by these immune reactions and by unusual cytotoxic leukotriene immune substances and increased numbers of CD8+

cytotoxic cells shown to circulate in CMT blood (7). These results demonstrate the relationship between the immune system and low fatty acids in CMT patients. The key omega-6 fatty acids, linoleic and arachidonic acids, appear to be diverted from blood stores for the formation of immunoregulatory prostaglandins and leukotrienes in CMT patients during this aberrent autoimmune process (3,5,7,10,11).

Altered immunity in CMT is consistent with the reported increase of CMT symptoms during the stress of pregnancy (12) and following trauma and operations (13). The findings of the pregnancy study are summarized in the following abstract from *Neurology* 1993; 43:2011-2016. "We report the obstetric complications and the influence of pregnancy and delivery in 21 Charcot-Marie-Tooth disease Type I (CMT I) patients with 45 gestations. Sixteen patients had subjective disabilities from childhood or youth, and five with late onset had subclinical CMT when they became pregnant. The rate of obstetric complications in the study group was in accordance with that of the normal population, and there was no deleterious effect on fetal outcome. Of the 21 participants, 38% (8 of 21) reported an exacerbation of CMT in at least one pregnancy. These patients noted increasing weakness in 81% (17 of 21) of their gestations. A temporary worsening occurred in 35% (6 of 17) of these pregnancies, and neurologic disabilities persisted after 65% of the deliveries (11 of 17). Patients who had pregnancy-associated progression in the first gestation (7 of 21) experienced similar deterioration in subsequent pregnancies (10 of 11), i.e., there is a high risk of recurrence of exacerbations. Four women, (19%) stated that their last deliveries were responsible for either an exacerbation or the onset of the neuropathy. The remaining nine patients (43%) denied any effect of their gestations on the progression of the neuropathy. Among the patients who had subjective disabilities from childhood or youth the risk of a noticeable exacerbation in at least one pregnancy was 50% (8 of 16) and affected

81% of their gestations (17 of 21), whereas there was no influence of pregnancy in the five patients with adult onset of CMT, although the first symptoms were noticed postpartum in two of them. Neither age at onset, age at delivery, interval between onset and delivery, or order or number of gestations are useful criteria for predicting a pregnancy-related progression of CMT I."

Genetic Counseling and the Implications of Chromosomal Tests

CMT historic genetic family trees can now be supplemented by definitive chromosomal tests for the presence of a duplicated, possibly defective, CMT gene on chromosome 17 (13,15). This test identifies a CMT locus characterizing CMT patients and carriers of CMT Type 1 A. The degree of gene duplication may indicate the general severity of symptoms, but this and other aspects of CMT variants are under intense study (see Genetics Chapter). The nature and expense of this genetic test should be evaluated carefully for the CMT family.

Personal factors must be considered before searching for the defective CMT gene. The knowledge of being an affected carrier or possibly becoming symptomatic in time may be emotionally detrimental or frightening to certain individuals. While medical heredity concepts must be translated into an understandable form for the CMT patient and family, it is also important to address the guilt and fears brought about by an "inherited condition." In addition, current medical ignorance about the CMT process should be acknowledged honestly to family members. In my experience, many patients detected a "hesitation" in their doctors when discussing CMT, brought about by this lack of knowledge, and misinterpreted it as the doctor's reluctance to "tell them the awful truth." Misunderstandings compound anxiety and fear in the CMT patient and family, and require reassurance and patience from the primary care physician. Positive statements such as "CMT can be lived with; it is not a fatal disease," are most helpful.

To establish good rapport, it is wise to share with CMT families these unknown elements of genetic research. In brief, they are 1) the location of all the CMT genes, 2) where and what the abnormal proteins of CMT are, 3) what determines penetrance of the defective genes, 4) what controls the genetic disease course, and lastly 5) whether and when there may be effective genetic techniques for prevention or treatment. Since CMT is not life-threatening and there is no treatment at present, many families may understandably reject the knowledge and expense of chromosome surveys until these can provide realistic therapeutic options.

Legal Aspects in CMT Disease

CMT families usually have intrafamilial examples of apparent and often major variations in clinical expression in the family members who presumably carry the same CMT gene. The natural CMT disease course is a slowly but irregularly progressive deterioration of peripheral motor and sensory functions (13). Although the disease is bilateral, there is often marked asymmetry in the clinical deficits of CMT patient limbs, as originally noted by Charcot, Marie, and Tooth. In addition, there may be short (weeks) or long (years) periods of exacerbation of the CMT disease. During exacerbation, the particular muscle or nerve area acutely involved in the pathologic process may be very painful with night cramping (13).

These aspects are very difficult or impossible to explain in terms of a purely genetic response. As a result, the patient's concern may lead to enrolling the legal system to determine whether work or other stresses may have augmented the CMT process. The primary caretaker will be expected to be an expert witness. A definite relationship between stress and physical deficiencies has not been demonstrated in CMT. This is a "gray" area, although it has been postulated that immunologic controls can affect genetic expression (14). Since the absolute answer is not yet known, testimony in court can be difficult for the medical professional. In contrast, if it can be emphasized by the medical caretaker that these changes are commonly found in CMT and a positive light placed on the future, grief and worry as well as legal expenses may be avoided.

Rules for CMT Patient Management

1. One primary health caretaker must take the responsibility for a positive, helpful LONG-TERM relationship with the CMT patient and family. On-going emotional support, simple explanations, and medical advice should be combined with suitable referrals described below.

2. A primary caretaker or neurologist needs to explain the CMT disease process to the patient and family, admitting honestly the limits of our current knowledge.

3. A neurologist may best be able to establish the correct CMT diagnosis using neurologic examinations, electromyographs, nerve conduction studies, and possibly chromosome tests.

4. A neurologist or primary care physician may participate in investigative studies and add new drugs or therapies as they become available.

5. For treatment of physical handicaps, referrals should include the services of the Muscular Dystrophy Clinic, orthopedic surgeons, podiatrists, physical and occupational therapists, physiatrists, and social workers.

6. The primary caretaker should provide information for healthful living: normal weight, adequate diet, avoidance of stress, and treatment of infections.

7. The primary caretaker should anticipate the possible development of decreased physical functions and/or help prevent school-initiated or work-de-

rived injuries by writing letters to school officials and by suggesting job counseling or obtaining job retraining for handicapped individuals.

8. The primary caretaker should address each new symptom of the CMT patient over time with new attention and concern, emphasizing a positive and cheerful outlook for the future to the CMT patient and family.

References:

1. Yao JK, Ellefson RD, Dyck PJ. Lipid abnormalities in hereditary neuropathy I Serum non-polar lipids. *J Neurol Sci* ; 29: 161-75, 1976.

2. Yao JK, Dyck PJ, Lipid abnormalities in hereditary neuropathy II. *J Neurol Sci* ; 36: 225-36, 1978.

3. Williams LL, O'Dougherty MM, Wright FS, Bobulski RJ, Horrocks LA. Dietary essential fatty acids, vitamin E, and Charcot-Marie-Tooth disease. *Neurology*; 36, 1200-05, 1986.

4. Williams LL O'Dougherty MM, Wright FS, Bobulski RJ, Horrocks LA. Essential fatty acid dietary addition in hereditary neuropathy. *Prog Lipid Res*; 25:607-10, 1986.

5. Williams LL, O'Dougherty MM, Wright FS, *et al.* Review: Effects of a dietary linoleic (omega-6) fatty acid and vitamin E supplementation on Type I CMT serum fatty acids and physical performance. In: Charcot Marie-Tooth Disorders: Pathophysiology, Molecular Genetics, and Therapy. R Lovelace and H Shapiro (eds), Alan Liss, New York, 1990: pp 403-7.

6. Williams LL , Wright FS. Arachidonic fatty acid in red blood cell membranes, lymphocytes, and cultured skin fibroblasts of dominant Charcot-Marie-Tooth syndrome. *J Neurol Sci* 1994 (in press).

7. Williams LL, Shannon BT, Wright FS. Circulating cytotoxic immune components in dominant Charcot-Marie-Tooth syndrome. *J Clin Immunol* ; 13: 389-96, 1993.

8. Williams LL. Pyruvate oxidation in Charcot-Marie-Tooth disease. *Neurology*; 29:1492-8, 1979.

9. Williams LL, Penn GM. Selective IgA deficiency in Charcot-Marie-Tooth disease. *Am J Clin Path;* 72: 800-6, 1979.

10. Williams LL, Shannon BT, O'Dougherty MM, Wright FS. Activated T-cells in T Type I Charcot-Marie-Tooth disease; evidence of immunologic heterogeneity. *J Neuroimmunol* ; 16: 317-330, 1987.

11. Williams LL, Kissel JT, Shannon BT, *et al.* Expression of Schwann cell and peripheral T-cells activation epitopes in hereditary motor and sensory neuropathy. *J Neuroimmunol*; 36:147-155, 1992.

12. Rudnik-Schoneborn S, Rohrig D, Nicholson G, Zerres K. Pregnancy and delivery in Charcot-Marie-Tooth disease Type I. *Neurology*; 43:2011-16, 1993.

13. Lupski JR, Garcia CA, Parry GJ, Patel PI. Charcot-Marie-Tooth polyneuropathy syndrome: clinical, electrophysiologic and genetic aspects. In: Current Neurology, S Appel (ed). Chicago, Mosby Yearbook 1991, pp 1-25.

14. Caskey CT. Presymptomatic diagnosis: A first step toward genetic health care. *Science*; 262:48-9, 1993.

15. Lupski JR, Wise CA, Kuwano A, *et al.* Gene dosage is a mechanism for Charcot-Marie-Tooth disease type 1A. *Nature Genetics*; 1:29-33, 1992.

Resources for the Charcot-Marie-Tooth Patient and Physician

The blood test for detecting the CMT IA gene found on chromosome 17 is available from **Athena Diagnositcs,** a subsidiary of Athena Neurosciences, Inc. Athena can be reached by calling Client Services at 1-800-394-4493. A physician must request the customized prepaid shipping kit for transport of the blood specimen to Athena. This kit contains specimen requirements and shipping/handling instructions. The cost of the test is $395.00. Please note: This test also detects Hereditary Neuropathy with Liability to Pressure Palsy (HNPP).

Also available is a blood test for detecting CMTX. Call an Athena Diagnsotics Client Services Representative for more information at 1-800- 394-4493.

- Athena Diagnostics
  Four Biotech Park
  377 Plantation Street
  Worcester, MA 01605
  Call 800-394-4493 for information on the CMT 1A DNA Testing Service (*exclusively* available from Athena Diagnostics).

The Charcot-Marie-Tooth Association (CMTA) has a program of education and support for the CMT patient and physician which includes a quarterly newsletter, patient handbooks, VCR tapes, conferences, and support groups. The CMTA Medical Advisory Board represents the CMT research and clinical communities. For further information contact:

- CMTA
  601 Upland Avenue
  Upland, PA 19015
  800-606-2682

The Muscular Dystrophy Association (MDA) will, upon referral, diagnose and evaluate CMT patients at no patient cost. They will provide an annual evaluation for physical therapy, occupational therapy, and respiratory therapy. For the informational brochure <u>MDA SERVICES For the Individual and Community</u>, contact:

- MDA
  3300 East Sunrise Drive
  Tucson, AZ 85718-3208
  602-529-2000

The Shriners' Hospitals will, at no cost, treat children from birth to 21 years of age. Their services include diagnosis, surgery, bracing, and physical/occupational therapies. For further information contact:

- Shriners' Hospitals for Crippled Children
  2900 Rocky Point Drive
  Tampa, FL 33607
  800-237-5055

The Easter Seal Society offers physical therapy, occupational therapy, and speech therapy to children and adults on an ability to pay basis. For further information contact:

- The National Easter Seal Society
  230 West Monroe Street, 18th Floor
  Chicago, IL 60606
  800-221-6827

Anesthesia and the CMT Patient

The following information is from a study done by Dr. Joseph Antognini, an anesthesiologist at the University of CA Davis Medical Center.

Dr. Antognini reviewed operative charts from 86 CMT patients on whom a total of 161 surgical procedures were performed. The conclusion of the study was, "the CMT patients evaluated in this survey appeared to tolerate anesthesia well. Although succinylcholine (SCH) has been considered to be contraindicated in this disease, no complications occurred from its use in these patients who had chronic symptoms. An acute exacerbation, however, might render SCH use inadvisable. Other risks, including sensitivity to neuromuscular blocking agents and malignant hyperthermia (MH), are probably minimal. The possibility of occult pulmonary dysfunction should be considered, but, in general, the anesthetic management in CMT can be adjusted to the needs of the individual patient." This article appeared in the Canadian Journal of Anesthesiology 39:pp 398-400, 1992. For a reprint of this article contact Dr. Joseph Antognini Dept. of Anesthesiology, U.C. Davis Medical Center 2315 Stockton Blvd. Sacramento CA 95817.

MEDICAL ALERT

Certain Drugs Toxic to the Peripheral Nervous System

This is a list of neurotoxic drugs which could be harmful to the CMT patient.

Adriamycin
Alcohol
Amiodarone
Chloramphenicol
Cis-platinum
Dapsone
Diphenylhydantoin
(Dilantin)
Disulfiram (Antabuse)
Glutethimide (Doriden)
Gold
Hydralazine (Apresoline)
Isoniazid (INH)
Mega Dose of Vitamin A
Mega Dose of Vitamin D
Mega Dose of Vitamin B_6
(Pyridoxine)
Metronidazole (Flagyl)
Nitrofurantoin
(Furadantin, Macrodantin)
Nitrous Oxide
(chronic repeated inhalation)
Penicillin
(Large IV doses only)
Perhexiline (Pexid)
Taxol
Vincristine

Lithium and Misomidazole can be used with caution.

Before taking any medication discuss it fully with your physician for possible side effects. 7/95

Reprinted with permission from the Charcot-Marie-Tooth Association.

Handbook Order Form

Name ____

Address ____
Street

____
City

____
State Zip Country

Please send _____ copies of the Physician's Handbook at $20.00 per copy in the U.S., $25.00 outside the U.S. (includes surface postage). Payment for foreign orders will be accepted by credit card, international money order or check drawn in U.S. dollars on a U.S. bank.

The total enclosed is $ _________ .

Payment (check one):

☐ Mastercard card # ____________________

☐ Visa expiration date: ____________________

☐ American Express

☐ check or money order ________________________
signature

Make checks payable to the Charcot-Marie-Tooth Association

Send Orders to: Charcot-Marie-Tooth Association
601 Upland Avenue,Upland, PA 19015

Index

E

F

G

H

I

K

M

N

T

V

W

X